Dr Nirdosh's
Anti-Ageing Secrets

Dr Nirdosh's Anti-Ageing Secrets

Dr Neetu Nirdosh

metro

Published by Metro Publishing
an imprint of John Blake Publishing Ltd
3 Bramber Court, 2 Bramber Road,
London W14 9PB, England

www.johnblakepublishing.co.uk

First published in paperback in 2010

ISBN: 978 1 84454 948 1

British Library Cataloguing-in-Publication Data:

A catalogue record for this book is available from the British Library.

Design by www.envydesign.co.uk

Printed in Great Britain by CPI Bookmarque, Croydon

1 3 5 7 9 10 8 6 4 2

Papers used by John Blake Publishing are natural, recyclable products made
from wood grown in sustainable forests. The manufacturing processes conform to
the environmental regulations of the country of origin.

ABOUT THE AUTHOR

Dr Nirdosh is a pioneer of London's Medical Anti-Ageing profession and she regularly instructs the media, magazine editors and directs beauty houses. As a celebrity beauty doctor, she has looked after scores of red-carpet stars. The exclusive Dr Nirdosh Anti-Ageing Clinic in London has been a private A-list haven for years, relied upon for the unique six-week anti-ageing plan and skin treatments. These are used daily by some of London's elite as their only anti-ageing regime.

She also established the first ever Anti-Ageing Fit Camp and is founder of DrNirdosh.com, the exclusive online health, beauty and anti-ageing store.

Dr Nirdosh combined modern science with new technologies and integrated 10 years of clinical research to formulate an elite range of anti-ageing skincare treatments and cosmetic youth pills that focus on reversing the causes of ageing by targeting deeper cellular levels of skin ageing that surgery cannot reach or repair. The Dr Nirdosh treatments work in conjunction with the four-step anti-ageing plan and are the only treatments to provide a complete head-to-toe anti-ageing blitz around the clock.

I dedicate this book to my dearest father who gave me the edge to get here, enabling me to strive towards success.

I am eternally grateful to my mother for moulding me from a youngster into the beauty doctor I am today and giving me the health knowledge not found in any text books!

Thanks to my agent and friend Mark Thomas for all his efforts with this book, unremitting support and sharing my visions!

Exceptional thanks to Answar Chay Mahmood. You make the impossible possible and your endless hours have been instrumental to the accomplishment of this book.

GLOSSARY OF TERMS

HGH	Human Growth Hormone
EIGR	Exercise Induced Growth Hormone Release
DOMS	Delayed Onset Muscle Soreness
EFAs	Essential Fatty Acids
EDJ	Epidermal Dermal Junction
HRT	Hormone Replacement Therapy
GHSs	Growth Hormone Secretagogues
OPCs	Oligomeric Proanthocyanidins
SOD	Superoxide Dismutase

Contents

Introduction

MANY A-LIST beauties and celebrities follow my revolutionary needle- and knife-free, all-natural 'face- and body-lift' plan to retain a younger, glowing face and sexier body.

As we age, the body's ability to remain young and sexy rapidly diminishes and this downward spiral becomes evident in wrinkles, dull, drooping skin and a soft, fat-ridden, out-of-shape body. My new miracle plan will help reverse your body's ageing process and recapture your youth in just six weeks. My plan is a six-week plan but my advice is to continue to follow it even after the six weeks are up. After six weeks, continue with the six-hour fasting gaps but introduce two treat meals per week. Within reason, eat whatever you like during these treat meals – knowing that you have these to look forward to will allow you to remain focused on your diet plan.

In this book, I finally reveal the vital medical components that will prepare your body to beat those ageing blues. I'll show you how to de-age your face and body in unison by using my unique exercise techniques, diet plan, supplements and skincare treatments. The special 'Nirdosh effect' will take your body from a degenerative, ageing state and transform it to a regenerative, anti-ageing condition.

Unlike many others in the industry, I am a proper doctor – fully trained in the NHS, with Bachelor of Medicine and Surgery degrees (MB CHB). My mother had worked as a beautician and dance teacher and my father was a mathematician, so the disciplines of both science and beauty have always been part of my background.

For six years, I trained at the University of Birmingham Medical School. I then worked around the clock for four years as a practising doctor in the Medical Admissions unit of an NHS Trust hospital where I dealt with patients suffering every imaginable type of illness and condition.

The Dr Nirdosh Anti-Ageing Plan was devised in my darkest hours as a junior doctor while fighting against the elements of long shifts, poor nutrition, sleep deprivation, depression and premature ageing. My hectic schedule as a medic meant that I had little time to look after myself and I became stuck in a depressive rut where life became a race against time and my health took a back seat.

From my youth I had always had a keen interest in the body's ageing process and, while at medical school, began researching how to prolong youth and concluded that there could be a link between growth hormones and prevention of ageing. Once I had qualified and started working as a junior doctor, I privately continued my investigative studies and, after years of efforts, unravelled my master anti-ageing plan. The plan was developed using intense medical research and collation of science, in particular endrocrinology, gerontology and geriatric medicine, sports medicine, human anatomical science, dermatology and neurological studies.

Led by my discovery that anti-ageing hormones are truly the magic bullet to youth, I'll show you how to reignite declining levels of this extraordinary, age-defying chemical. My medically developed plan boosts skin-cell immunity and trains your face and body to win the fight against ageing.

Anti-ageing hormones are the body's youth messengers. Over time, levels are rapidly lost, exposing a host of problems, including thinning skin, weight gain and invisible internal damage. Much is easily missed by the naked eye: deterioration of lean muscle, accumulation of fat, weakened bones, as well as far more serious medical conditions, such as heart disease and impaired brain acuity.

This book reveals how to use special anti-ageing, hormone-boosting technology and skin immunity rechargers to evade the ageing process. Indeed, you can actually programme your system to destroy unwanted invaders and instigate speedy repair of an unfit, unhealthy body complete with wrinkles, wounds and age scars.

As the doctor and pioneering anti-ageing specialist behind many famous red-carpet bodies, I promise to share with you all my A-list anti-ageing secrets and provide a prescription for a younger face, sexier body, rejuvenated sex drive and more exciting life in just six weeks! This powerful plan puts decades of youth back into your system and, as you'll soon discover, it isn't at all complicated.

So, read on and learn how to undo ageing using my specialist four-step plan of nutrition, workouts, skincare and supplements designed to enhance skin immunity and activate anti-ageing hormones – those vital compounds lost with age and responsible for all things old.

Chapter 1
Dr Nirdosh Prescribes Everlasting Youth

MANY OF YOU may already be ageing faster than you thought possible and perhaps you fear that the ageing process is taking control of you. But forget that fear: you have in your hands the only anti-ageing medical book that can put you back in control. Follow the Dr Nirdosh Anti-Ageing Plan and you'll discover how to make your face look younger and achieve the ultimate youthful body.

Many A-list celebrities and socialites are secretly using my plan on a daily basis to turn back the clock. This unique prescription is a needle-free solution to bring stunning results in just a few weeks for anyone, of any age. Instead of cursing yet another facial wrinkle as you look in the mirror each day, being on the plan ensures that you will relish waking up – you'll learn to love your face as your wrinkles soften and become less apparent.

As your face starts to look decades younger, your body will simultaneously be transformed. When you look at yourself naked in that mirror, no longer will you see horrid fatty rolls and sagging skin staring back at you. Instead, your dream body will soon begin to take shape right in front of your very eyes. You'll see a lean, fat-free and perfectly formed physique so defined and sexy that it definitely demands a second look. At the same time, your whole body will unravel the ageing process still more with the return of your sex drive. Your libido levels will go through the roof as you discover a sex drive you never knew existed or rediscover the one of yesteryear.

My powerful anti-ageing plan works directly on the major concerns, such as thinning skin, lines, wrinkles, a sagging neck and weight gain, plus invisible internal damage – much of it easily missed by the naked eye. This includes deterioration of lean muscle, accumulation of fat, bone weakening, as well as serious medical conditions, including heart disease, diabetes and impaired brain acuity.

There are two ways to age: the first gives a youthful face and body, sex appeal, longevity and confidence; with the second come age-related illnesses that make you feel and look old. You never had the option before, but with the Dr Nirdosh Anti-Ageing Plan you do now, and I urge you to choose it!

HOW MY PLAN WORKS

Meticulously developed over a decade to provide the body with the necessary components to defy and counteract ageing, for the first time ever the Dr Nirdosh Anti-Ageing Plan gives users – both male and female – a realistic, revolutionary needle- and knife-free face- and body-lift. In just six weeks, the whole body can be transformed, internally and externally. My plan targets the core areas responsible for keeping your body young and that's why it's more successful than any other.

The principle is simple: the Dr Nirdosh Anti-Ageing Plan refuses to allow the body to age. As anti-ageing hormone levels decline internally, the plan kicks into action to ensure your body tops them right up again to fight back. So, how is this possible? These hormones are the key components we need to stay looking young. With age, they decline, but, through reigniting waning levels of this extraordinary age-defying chemical, the face and body can be trained to win the battle against ageing.

The principal anti-ageing hormone is the Human Growth Hormone (HGH), the superpower of anti-ageing hormones, and one which I will go on to talk about throughout the book. Other anti-ageing hormones enhanced on my plan are:

- Dehydroepiandrosterone – this functions both as an anti-ageing hormone and also as a precursor to make other hormones
- Thyroid Hormone – a metabolic hormone
- Oestrogen – female sex hormone
- Progesterone – female sex hormone
- Testosterone – male sex hormone also present in females (see chapter 11)
- Melatonin – sleep hormone
- Endorphins – feelgood hormones

Through the powers of body manipulation alone, without injections or surgery, anti-ageing hormones may be naturally reinjected into the face and body with my four-step plan of unique exercise techniques, diet, anti-ageing supplements and skincare treatments. In turn, your body will be freed from an accelerated state of ageing, instantly positioning it in a regenerative age-defiant state as it quickly starts to refuel itself with the lost anti-ageing hormones necessary to produce a natural, needle-free lift. The benefits of the plan, as detailed below, are truly astonishing.

The Natural Anti-Ageing Face-Lift will give you:
- A natural, younger-looking and more uplifted face
- Thicker, plumper facial skin
- Fewer fine lines and wrinkles
- Diminished crow's feet and eye bags
- Tighter neck and jowls; also tighter facial skin with less sag
- Radiant, glowing skin
- Finally, stronger, more tactile skin – quite simply, a whole new you!

The Natural Anti-Ageing Body-Lift provides:
- A beautiful, lean, and fat-free body that looks decades younger
- Slender, more defined thighs and hips
- Cellulite-free legs without lumpy, orange-peel skin
- A washboard stomach
- Shapely arms with muscle definition
- A gorgeously uplifted, pert bottom
- Finally, a higher-lifted bust and deeper cleavage line – in all, a sexy, curvaceous, tauter frame.

So, follow my plan to reverse the ageing process and reap these advantages:

- The body is encouraged to live up to two decades longer
- Improved heart function, so lowering the risk of cardiovascular disease
- Enhanced muscle tissue in the whole body, producing a firmer frame
- Elevated brain function, encouraging a better memory and sharper cognitive actions
- A halt to bone demineralisation and osteoporosis
- Confidence is boosted and depression wiped clean away
- Amplified libido – feel your sex drive skyrocket!
- Immunity is reinforced to fend off illnesses better.

THE NIRDOSH SCIENCE

During my years studying medicine at university, I was fascinated to discover that the body can resist the process of ageing. This developed into a passion for greater knowledge of the process and led me to discover the real cause of ageing. My enthusiasm went back as far as the days when I toured the UK as a professional dancer in my youth. From the age of four, I was performing tap and ballet.

In those days, little information existed on how to maintain stamina, youthfulness and general good health, so I had to teach myself the right foods for optimum wellbeing. My mother had always insisted on feeding us fresh and nutritious foods and our meals at home were very healthy, with the kitchen being the hub of family life. My mother taught me that eating fruit and vegetables (especially in their raw state), low-fat milk and nuts rich in special oils would protect my skin and prevent lines and wrinkles from developing. She drummed into me that what I ate early on in life would benefit me in years to come. Indeed, I was the only girl at school in my class who shunned crisps and chocolate, instead opting for a daily lunch of six tomatoes, half a cucumber, a raw carrot and a pint of milk. Although the other pupils laughed at me, I knew they were eating foods that would slow down their performance and make them fat and lethargic. Even in kids, the body must work hard to break down the sugary calories contained in junk food. In the long term, their health would suffer because the foods they were eating conflicted with the body's balance and so it reacted in turn by releasing insulin and cortisol, the bad ageing hormones linked to unhealthy foods.

So, what exactly causes ageing? At university, I questioned this further and started to unravel the major contributory factors in destroying youth. Most importantly, I established that ageing is a disease but it can be treated: it is a multi-faceted, chronic process that causes our organs, tissues and cells to progressively lose function. Eventually, this leads to numerous illnesses, among them heart disease, cancer, osteoporosis, diabetes, infections, loss of agility, postural problems and deterioration of the brain.

External age damage becomes apparent in the face with the onset of wrinkles, thin, drooping skin, crow's feet and age spots. Internally, however, something far more serious occurs: muscle tissue deterioration, loss of body tone and facial firmness. The key culprits are hormones. Throughout life, the body experiences a massive change in hormonal activity. Good anti-ageing hormones are already present in our bodies, but levels diminish rapidly, thanks to everyday lifestyle choices such as a poor diet, late nights, smoking, excessive alcohol, lack of exercise, dehydration and stress. All these trigger the release of bad ageing hormones, thus causing a series of negative catabolic breakdown reactions that leave the body in a progressively more fragile state as the bad hormones override the good ones. Prolonged bouts of such a negative cycle are responsible for your current health, body shape and facial structure. This is the ageing process at its rawest.

Just a quick word about the link between stress and ageing. Stress causes anti-ageing hormones to diminish and instead instigates a surge of cortisol in the body. Cortisol is a stress hormone normally released during the 'fight and flight' reaction, placing the body in a high state of alert. It increases the heart rate, enhances brain-to-muscle co-ordination, stimulates the mind, raises blood pressure and generally has catabolic breakdown effects. In small doses it is protective but chronic release can cause insulin resistance and predisposition to obesity by enhancing fat storage.

Often, we do nothing and accept ageing as a normal transition in life that we must experience. Having learned as a child that if you take care of your body then it has the tools it needs to implement positive changes, I have never accepted this. Indeed, if we block the age-inflicting hormones, this negative reaction cannot occur. Research has led me to conclude that the way to fight the ageing process is to send a surge of powerful, anti-ageing hormones back into the body to overrule the ageing ones. If you do this, you can slow down – and even reverse – the ageing process.

The real test happened when I became a Bachelor of Medicine and Surgery and started my clinical rotations in NHS hospitals. Non-stop, ninety-hour weeks as a junior doctor really took their toll and bad habits quickly became the norm as I ate processed snacks, sugary rubbish and fat-laden foods. During this time, I never drank water, exercise was a thing of the past and I gained a horrid, podgy stomach. Frequently, I had to do late nights and suffered sleep deprivation, with many of my shifts way beyond the call of duty. I had fallen into a trap and was experiencing firsthand premature, rapid ageing.

Fine lines were fast developing around my face, I had puffy, swollen baggy eyes and dry and scaly eczematous skin, plus the excess weight had covered my legs with cellulite. In my late twenties, I had already started to see grey hairs. This *had* to change!

From my research, I understood that ageing is a disease that can be treated and so I decided that now was the time to put my age-reversal plan into action. I wanted to restore a younger body and line-free face and I knew that I could achieve this by introducing anti-ageing hormones into my body to end the ageing process.

Using scientific research and medical expertise, plus my life experiences and passion, I created the revolutionary Dr Nirdosh Four-Step Plan – a foolproof system to give anyone a younger face and body. In order to harness the body's ability to manufacture anti-ageing hormones and resist further ageing, four doctor-developed disciplines are needed:

- Hormone-inducing exercises
- Eating plans
- Skincare treatments
- Anti-ageing supplements.

Once I introduced the plan into my life, the results were mind-blowing. Instantly, my face started to look less haggard, the lines and bags under my eyes disappeared. My body looked so different and – dare I say it –sexy, as I lost all the fat and couldn't wait to show off my new bikini body. The facial skin became far more lifted and I looked much younger.

My colleagues had never seen such a drastic change in just six weeks. While they stayed looking the same or even slightly older, I was looking younger. They asked if I'd had cosmetic surgery on my face and my body. By then, I had lost nearly three stone and the squidgy, soft body and bulging belly I once had were now replaced by a tight, sexy, muscular frame. The doctors I worked with asked me to reveal my plan so they could take it up and reverse their own ageing problems.

What they hadn't realised was that the anti-ageing hormones manufactured by me in my own body from the Four-Step Plan were counteracting ageing to make me look young again. Through the plan, I had replenished these hormones and not allowed my body to age. After that I continued with the plan without stopping and today I am regularly mistaken for a girl in her early twenties, even though I am actually in my late thirties!

NATURE'S ENGINEERING

On the Four-Step Plan, we help the body reproduce anti-ageing hormones and replenish declining levels to make it look young and beautiful again as follows:

- My exclusive exercises work by releasing anti-ageing hormones back into the body. Amazingly, the workouts last just 20 minutes each, but transform your body by unleashing a surge of hormones through a series of special movements.

- These hormones flood your body with the chemicals necessary to instigate regrowth, redevelopment, youth and beauty. This switches you back into a regenerative mode rather than a dangerous, degenerative one.

- The body no longer accepts that it is ageing and instead uses the new top-up hormones to reverse damage, thus healing and enabling it to remain ageless.

- My plan teaches you to eat yourself younger. The right foods include youth-enhancing nutrients and activate a special gene that helps to block ageing. Correct nutrition can help trigger the anti-ageing hormones.

- The next step is a skincare prescription of anti-ageing treatments. Using dedicated treatments for your exact skin type and age profile makes your face look much younger, allowing a full course of age-defying nutrients to repair the outer layer of skin that displays the signs of ageing.

- A prescription of specialised anti-ageing supplements is the

final step. You will consume vital anti-ageing supplements –
or, as I term them, youth pills – so age damage to the inner
layer of skin is treated head-on. This provides your face and
body with what they need to become youthful again and
prevent the external signs
of ageing.

Without dangerous chemicals or risky cosmetic surgery, we will
reinject anti-ageing hormones into the body. In fact, surgery is
probably the worst way to tackle ageing – outwardly, you may
appear young, but, inside, you still age at the same rate.

LIFE BEGINS AT 50

Most people believe we are conditioned to age and as such should
accept it as the inevitable. This preconception is currently going
through a dramatic change, however, and is now the view of the
minority. The world no longer obsesses purely about health and
all aspects related to the ageing process, such as heart disease,
strokes, obesity and diabetes; today youth and beauty are almost
as important, vanity more relevant than ever. In adopting the
anti-ageing lifestyle revealed within these pages, you really can
determine your ageing destiny. I'll provide you with the tools to
evolve and adapt youthfully.

Celebrities have taken stock. Let me mention a few names:
Madonna, Sigourney Weaver, Susan Sarandon and Sharon Stone.
What if I were to tell you that the one thing these iconic women
have in common is their age? They are all over 50 and they don't
look it, let alone act it. None of these stars shows any sign of

slowing down, quite the opposite, in fact. Most are in the prime of their careers with lovers or husbands half their age so life *can* begin at 50, but only for those who take action.

Knowing this, why do many of us assume, when we hit the big five-o, that our body's ability to act young, sexy and ageless will disappear altogether? Why are there such different attitudes towards ageing? Simply because the celebrities themselves are fully aware of the power of the human body and how it can be programmed with the right disciplines to reverse ageing processes and repair damage. They have the secret information and now you too have the anti-ageing secrets in your hands. No longer can you use the excuse that they are rich and famous, with the best doctors to guide them.

As your personal celebrity doctor, I will help you become young again. Follow my revolutionary plan and I promise you will look younger and trimmer – you'll also be sexier and live longer. As an additional bonus, your libido will soar, as a big part of the plan boosts your sex hormones, more of which later. Younger and sexier... what are you waiting for?

Chapter 2
The Ageing Process

THE PREMISE OF ageing is simple: as you grow older, you start to age – it's natural. Yet beautiful people seem to age better than others and, if you're one of the lucky few, you too can boast that the angel of beauty has been good to you and helped you defy ageing.

Do you believe what you've just read? If so, you are not alone – most men and women of a certain age openly admit that the issue of ageism is something they have been faced with at some stage in their lives. Normally, this is in their late twenties when they start to experience the first real signs of ageing. What tends to follow is a series of failed ventures to regain youth, whether cosmetic surgical intervention or topical face masks that promise younger skin, the latest age-reversing gizmo or even the sexual conquest of a younger suitor. However, eventually, they conclude that ageing is a natural process, one they should learn to accept and embrace, and some men and women are naturally more attractive than others. So, are they right?

The sad thing is that we are clearly a generation with our hearts set on clinging desperately on to our youth and those early years. Often we fail miserably and revert to the same point of view as our parents who liked to say, 'One day, you'll look old and wrinkly like me, so get used to it!' But they were wrong then and it is still untrue now. Accept it and you've just bought into an old wives' tale. Once and for all, this revolutionary book will blow that myth right out of the water.

You're about to implement life-changing principles and discover that ageing really is just for those who choose to do so. With the Dr Nirdosh Anti-Ageing Plan comes the option of welcoming a youth that lasts decades longer. The amazing thing about the plan is that it's never too late – you can begin at any age and get incredible results. How is all that possible? Well, let's look at the ageing process in more detail to understand why.

WHY WE AGE

As babies we are all born equal, with a neutral platform: this is the point at which the body equips you with its major quality. This alone is nature's most potent anti-ageing cure. It's the one trait that has doctors and scientists throughout the world pumping billions of pounds into research to find a way for us to stay young. So, what is the singular most important trait in the body? In a word: regeneration.

When we are toddlers, the human body's capabilities are totally different from those when we pass through puberty and enter adulthood. The body's ability to acquire youth is priceless and plentiful, achieved through its own anti-ageing capabilities for that regeneration.

Throughout life, our bodies progressively change. Drastic transformations turn us from being a baby into a teenager, into a young adult and then we become fully fledged adults. The biggest asset and the real difference between a younger body and that of an adult is that, during our younger years, the body rapidly grows stronger day by day and seems to glow in its new demure posture, confidence and sexual attractiveness. It's a great time for the body as it develops youth and agility.

From then on, the adult body is not composed in this way. Instead, it weakens as the years go by. There's a constant need to engage in the latest diet or exercise trend just to keep on feeling young, or at least to attempt to do so. In contrast, the body of a teen simply wakes up, eats, doesn't have to go to the gym, goes to bed and wakes up stronger. The saying 'Eat, drink and be merry' might have been written for teens because it's an adage universally followed by them. Wouldn't you love a body like that, one that grows more powerful and ever younger?

As adults, we reach a certain point where the body becomes affected by the everyday vices we engage in. 'Eat, drink and be merry' should have a second part attached to it: gain weight, become ill, continue like that and die! The reason why this sudden change occurs is because the body no longer becomes progressively stronger on a daily basis. Instead, it undergoes the one thing we all do our best to defy: ageing.

The process of ageing slowly takes the human body down a slippery road that leads to the negative physical and mental changes experienced by us all. What is the reason for this? In a word, degeneration: instead of rebuilding itself with health and vitality, in this state the body begins to break down.

Many people are under the mistaken impression that youth is a phase in our lives that comes and goes. The real problem is that the body's ability to regenerate simply disappears and, with it, so does our youth. So, is this a genetic thing? Do some people have the potential to regenerate and go on feeling and looking younger for longer than others? Perhaps you have friends and family members who look better than you. Are glamorous-looking celebrities gifted with better chromosomes than the rest of us? The answer to all these questions is a big NO!

In the next six weeks, you'll learn why this is a myth as you embark on my anti-ageing plan, and while everyone else comments on how amazing you look. If you want to be mean, tell them it's purely down to your family's good genes! The reality is that genetics have very little to do with the way we age. Of course, there's no denying they have some impact on how we look and develop, but this is just a tiny amount, perhaps about 20 per cent. The remaining 80 per cent is an individual quality because the current image of your body is down to you alone.

Old wives' tales were fine in yesteryear when technology was unable to prove otherwise. As a celebrity anti-ageing doctor regularly called on to reinvent and reverse ageing in my clients, however, I have researched and taken advantage of the resources available through medical intervention to explode the myth about ageing. In the process, I've discovered the necessary tools for you to become young again.

THE BIG MISCONCEPTION ABOUT AGEING

Now you know that ageing is not so simple, the next misconception for me to blow apart is that we cannot reverse it. You now know that ageing is a by-product of degeneration, the loss of which explains why the body progressively ages. What if we were to boost the body with something to make it really young again, so that it could take on the same traits – a body that could defy ageing and grow younger by the day? That's exactly what this book is about to do, to show you a scientific way to create regeneration naturally, something that has never been done before.

This method of mine was at first used by celebrities alone, but there's no reason why it should remain a secret – I want it to work for you, too. Rest assured there's no need to take part in any kind of risky surgical procedure or to jump on to a freaky machine. With the Dr Nirdosh Anti-Ageing Plan, your body has the power to regenerate and reintroduce youth.

The medical profession itself is a major culprit in this whole muddled fiasco: some doctors are constantly on the lookout for newer, more bizarre procedures as the answer to regaining youth. In doing so, they veer off in completely the wrong direction. They have never made the correct correlation about the underlying reasons why we age. Indeed, when I flagged this up at university, it was brushed aside and ignored.

What so many of my fellow medics fail to see is that the ageing process is simply the adult body's inability to regenerate, which means the whole focus should be around the possibility of regenerating our systems. I have created this plan to allow the regeneration process to be reignited and that's why so many celebrities today rely on it to make them feel good and look decades younger. My scheme has the additional benefit of increased longevity, giving them back an extra 20 years of life by reversing their age clock. Of course, this is something that surgery could never achieve.

Regeneration acts like a universal switch. Just turn it on and the body can be programmed to become younger, more beautiful and sexier still.

THE AGEING CULPRITS

So what actually causes the ageing process that we are constantly fighting? Does the body deteriorate naturally, or are we responsible for this through our everyday lifestyles? Now we'll take a look at some of the major causes of ageing.

Smoking

Let's be clear, inhaling tobacco causes wrinkles and quickly ages the face. It's one of the biggest skin and body age-accelerators, yet it's hard to believe that nearly a million people each year light up for the first time. Quite alarming when you consider the number of warnings on cigarette packs, which say smoking kills.

Astonishingly, this deadly habit is now just as common as it was 10 years ago. Many people start smoking in their teenage years, some even as young as twelve and the only real change is that there now seem to be more female smokers than male. Indeed, statistics prove nicotine is more addictive for women than men, although both sexes often regret this habit in their later years.

Cigarettes damage the skin and cause fast wrinkle development, especially around the mouth. Excessively pursing of the lips to take a puff draws in tobacco smoke and toxins that litter the area around the mouth with perioral lines (permanent smoking age lines). What's more, smoking rapidly depletes levels of vitamins A and C in the body, causing the skin to lose its ability to remain plump, radiant and firm. Instead, it starts to sag and form jowls.

One of the major problems with smoking is that it breaks down collagen, something no man or woman wants because it furthers skin sagging beyond the face to the arms and neck. The damage to the face is severe, yet this is minimal compared to the body because smoking causes serious medical illnesses, such as cancer, strokes and heart attacks, and takes years off your life expectancy. It also blocks oxygen and nutrient access to the skin by restricting blood flow in capillaries. Really, this is a no-no when it comes to reversing the ageing process. Then there's the bad breath and the smell on your clothes.

If you're struggling to kick the habit, visit the NHS Stop Smoking website (www.smokefree.nhs.uk), where there are government programmes set up especially to help you.

Alcohol

Drinking alcohol in vast quantities causes skin to age rapidly, as the high sugar content enhances wrinkle formation. More dangerous still, though, is that alcohol ages the brain.

Today, women more than men seem to be in denial about the amount of alcohol they consume. It's common for people to admit, 'I consume a bottle of wine with a good meal,' without actually realising they have a problem that is spiralling out of control.

Amid all the potential addiction issues, alcohol is a fast track to ageing badly and the damage is more than just skin-deep. The brain is heavily affected by drink as it speeds up loss of brain cells and eats away at the nervous system, which in turn impairs judgement and memory. Another problem is that alcohol is a depressant. In fact, it instigates depression and can even be the cause of a deep clinical depression. Further complications stemming from this include diabetes, liver disease, ulcers, cancers and heart attacks. Since alcohol masks pain through its anaesthetic effect, it can hide the symptoms of a heart attack and this is dangerous in itself.

Don't forget that alcohol is also loaded with calories. A glass of wine or champagne can contain anything upwards of 100 calories, while a pint of lager weighs in at about 200 calories. Just a few drinks in the evening can take you way over your recommended daily calorie allowance and the extra sugar in the alcohol will eventually be stored as fat. The sugar in booze will also wreak havoc on the skin, as the glucose latches on to collagen fibres and disrupts the collagen, a vital skin protein that keeps the face firm. Drinking excessive amounts of alcohol also causes inflammatory skin flare-ups including acne, rosacea and broken thread veins.

A big confidence loss associated with alcohol is that it kills your levels of sexual libido. Although small amounts may lead to a loss of inhibition, large quantities decrease sexual desire and the ability to perform.

Do bear in mind, however, that we are talking about heavy drinking here, not your run-of-the-mill glass of wine. Small amounts of alcohol can have great benefits and are recommended as part of this anti-ageing plan!

Here are some tips to help you keep your alcohol intake under control:

- Alternate your drinks – have an alcoholic one followed by a non-alcoholic one.
- Set your limit before you go out – and stick to it!
- Sip your drink slowly, don't guzzle it down.
- On a night out, distract yourself from drinking with other activities such as chatting and dancing.
- Always go for a small glass size.
- Don't start the night out by drinking at home – wait until you get there.
- Remember that the recommended weekly alcohol allowances are 14 units for women and 21 units for men (one glass of wine or half a pint of beer is equal to one unit).
- Don't forget that, on the Dr Nirdosh Plan, you are allowed a certain amount of red wine!

Sleep

Lack of sleep causes rapid ageing and the consequence of sleep deprivation shows itself on your face in the form of bags under the eyes, wrinkly skin, loss of skin firmness and a sallow complexion. The body relies on sleep for rest and recovery because during this phase it works hard to repair damage. If you rob it of one of its natural repair processes, you will increase the speed at which you age.

Lack of sleep doesn't only cause external problems that manifest themselves on your face, it also deepens internal ageing. This is a serious issue, which in turn elevates the risk of diabetes, memory loss, an unstable digestive system and obesity. Since the face bears the brunt of the symptoms caused by a lack of sleep, you should aim to get a good seven to eight hours each night if you intend to go on looking youthful.

Nutrition

Common sense prevails when food is related to ageing. Consuming products laden with fat, sugar and heavy in calories not only to leads to weight gain, but also causes premature ageing. The right foods can help your skin become young again, that's why they are so central to the process of anti-ageing.

Green vegetables and leafy salads contain the winning components: high-strength vitamins and antioxidants, which encourage the body to beat the ageing process. Oily fish, nuts and avocadoes are all rich in omega 3 and omega 6 essential fatty acids which make up our cell walls. They help to smooth lines and wrinkles by releasing moisture into dry skin. Sugary products, however, break down vital skin collagen, instigating the wrinkle-formation process. Habitually eating these bad foods leads to heart disease and rapid weight gain. The body's ability to use those junk calories as high-energy fuel is diminished because they only provide a quick boost; this is rarely sustained and is then followed by sudden low-energy levels. This unpleasant cycle causes bingeing and provokes a desire to eat more fast food, which, in turn, keeps the body in a premature ageing cycle.

The face and body need certain nutrients to help them repair themselves and this includes the right antioxidants, vitamins and minerals to aid growth, healing and recovery, which keep vital organs such as the skin agile and youthful. If we don't consume the right nutrients and these are instead compensated with the wrong type of junk-related calories, with no nourishing vitamins, minerals or antioxidants, then the body can develop diabetes, skin ageing and even a time-ticking heart attack.

More people than ever are being diagnosed as morbidly obese. It's a medical time bomb waiting to explode and one the nation has yet to defeat. Mortality, quality of life and skin condition are all linked to what you eat. In fact, life expectancy can drop by up to two or three decades if you continue to consume the wrong things. At the very least, your skin will lose its firmness and become saggy.

Exercise

A dormant body that gets no exercise is probably the biggest contributory factor to ageing. If you never do any kind of physical activity, then your face and body will soon start to look much older. Done correctly, the Dr Nirdosh Exercise Plan will provide the body with a rush of endorphins, adrenaline, growth hormone and testosterone, which have the combined effect of boosting energy and confidence and lifting the mood.

As the muscles lose their rigidity, your face begins to droop. Chances are, you will look older than your actual age. At the same time, your body starts to fall apart, with the development of bingo wings under the arms, a slackening chest, turkey neck, limp backside, fatty stomach and hideous jowls to boot. Need I say more?

If you fail to exercise, the body's metabolism also changes and you become prone to weight gain and open the gate to illnesses. Exercise keeps your immunity levels high and gives you a stronger body that is in good shape to fend off diseases, including ageing. As you enhance muscle tissue and your body becomes programmed to produce higher quantities of protein, these work to fight infection.

When you are ill, the body turns to special proteins (antibodies) to fend off foes. The problem is that they are made up of proteins, so, if you haven't built up a sufficient number of them, your body is less able to fight illnesses. Exercise achieves more than just weight loss, it's also a major anti-ageing heavyweight.

Sun Damage

With all the lethal health dangers of sun damage reported each holiday season, it's amazing that so many of us want to achieve the look of sun gods and goddesses. Since there are so many fake tanning creams around, I can't understand the logic of anyone choosing to tan under a machine that zaps you with radiation and ages you in the most dangerous way possible.

The sun is hugely powerful – it's our natural light source and keeps us alive. However, it's also one of the biggest age-accelerators. The brightest star harms the body in two ways:

- Skin collagen and elasticity is slowly demolished so you look wrinkled and leathery, like a reptile. Synthesis of new collagen is also impaired.
- Insufficient UV protection can lead to skin cancer depending on your skin colour and the amount of melanin or colour pigment it contains. The history of sun ageing normally follows a pattern: the lighter your skin tone, the more likely you are to suffer sun-induced age damage.

Age damage symptoms include wrinkles, age spots, freckles, fine lines, spider veins, sagging, deep creases, change in moles, rough skin and sometimes ultimately skin cancer. People often wonder how come they've suddenly got these symptoms; what they've forgotten or perhaps don't know is that, although the results of sun damage don't show until later years, the symptoms develop underneath the skin from early on.

Ensure you seek medical advice if you notice any skin changes such as new moles (or changes in the size or shape of existing moles), especially if they have an irregular outline, crust or bleed. Other skin changes that require immediate medical attention include skin growths, rashes and sunburn that won't heal. Spending a lot of time in intense sun can be dangerous, particularly if you have pale skin. Fairer skin contains less melanin (the pigment which acts as the skin's natural sunscreen, helping to absorb UV rays and prevent deeper penetration). Always make sure you wear a sunscreen too.

Having said all this, it is important to remember that, without some exposure to the sun, we couldn't survive. Sun enables the skin to produce vitamin D, which is needed for calcium and phosphate to be absorbed properly. The vitamin itself plays an important role in helping to control the rate of cell turnover, which can be important in protecting against certain cancers such as breast and colon cancer. Research has shown that exposure of just 15 minutes per day can be enough for the skin to produce its daily requirement of vitamin D. Long-term sun scarcity can lead to a shortfall of vitamin D that can in turn cause complications such as brittle bones.

Sun lovers don't notice any real change in their skin at the time that it occurs because nothing is visible to the naked eye. This encourages them to deem themselves immune to damage and therefore ignore UV protection.

When it comes to premature ageing, over-zealous exposure to the sun is a serious concern and often those who claim to have led a sun-kissed existence in some foreign location when they were young have deep-set wrinkles, hyperpigmentation and lines over their faces, arms, legs and body. Faced with the bright rays, good-quality UV protection must always be applied. Choose a broad-spectrum cream that safeguards the body against the environment's UVA and UVB rays and, for your own sake, please be aware that, even on dull days, UV protection should still be applied because clouds won't block radiation.

Stress

The world we live in is full of stress. Mundane tasks such as going to the supermarket can cause hassle, as can working for hours longer than intended, even meeting friends. But is it really bad for us to endure so much stress?

Stress is something that every human being faces at some point in his or her life. The trick is to minimise the amount of time the body remains in a stressed-out state – not only is long-term stress dangerous for the mind and body, but it's also one of the undercover ageing culprits that can make you look decades older than your real age.

Stress is indeed a major cause of premature ageing. If you don't believe me, just look at previous presidents, prime ministers and world leaders. Mostly, they enter the public arena with a spark of youth. Just four years on and often they look as if they've gained 20 years. The cause of this rapid ageing is stress.

Stress causes long-term expression lines on the face. When the skin is young and tactile, the face quickly bounces back into place, but, as the skin loses its youthfulness and starts to age, it loses the ability to spring back and expression lines turn to permanent age lines. The most common of these are forehead frown lines and crow's feet around the eyes. It's a difficult process to eliminate expression lines because you may not be aware that you are screwing up your face and so causing them. If you continue, they will become the profile of your face and the way other people see you.

The lines caused by ageing lead people to look for solutions in interventions such as Botox or face-lift surgery. At my clinic, I see people all the time who've been down the route of injectables and face-lifts. They want to look younger but soon realise that an injection is not the answer – especially when it goes wrong! These external procedures also do nothing to combat internal stress or slow down the ageing process – and, more importantly, we still do not know the long-term health implications of Botox and dermal fillers.

The fact that stress ages us internally affects the functioning of the mind and body by placing it in a cycle of anxiety. When this happens, the body reacts by trying to defend itself from what it fears is the approaching danger. Immediately it goes into the 'fight or flight' reaction, which is a natural defence mechanism. This is not a good thing at all – it means the body is now releasing all the chemicals that fast-forward ageing. If you remain in a high state of stress over a constant period of time, your body will show the signs of ageing in many ways, including hair thinning and loss, dermatitis and eczema, fine lines, wrinkles, high blood pressure and even heart attack, depressive moods and recurrent illnesses.

To counter this, you must quickly learn how to handle the stress and take up measures to protect yourself. Try exercise, meditation, taking up yoga, special breathing techniques and regularly look for a chance to laugh! All these solutions instantly bring down stress levels and make us feel happier. Also, be aware that you need to try to stop yourself making facial expressions such as frowning or squinting. Taking these steps will make you feel younger, more confident and in control of yourself.

THE AGEING DISEASE

So far, I have gone through all the factors that cause us to age. Now it's time for me to give you a new perspective on ageing, to make you think about the problem in a way you might never have done before. I'm about to reveal one more major ageing culprit that goes unmentioned in most other books: it's the special ageing criminal that we never take into account when we talk about the things that make us older: the need to treat ageing as a disease. For the main ageing culprit is this illness itself.

Losing your youth and becoming older causes the body to encounter chronic damage. This may seem obvious, but do not be fooled. Asked what causes you to age, the chances are that you would never mention ageing itself but instead might have opted for any of the above answers, such as smoking, the sun or junk food.

The missed ability to see ageing in this way is one of the reasons why we all age as we do. If we don't recognise it, then we don't do anything about it. To most people, including doctors and scientists, this is the real issue: it's not natural for us to regard ageing as a disease in itself, but rather we see it as a transition of life that just happens. Baloney! The premise that ageing kills youth is only true if you choose to believe it. My book will blow this thought right out of the water!

So, now you know all the major ageing culprits. The factors I have mentioned are collectively known as 'environmental ageing', a force that works to destroy your defence barriers against ageing. If you don't take action, then you'll continue on the road to destruction: your face will age, your body become out of shape and ridden with fat, you'll lose your sex drive, as well as the flexibility in your joints, and your internal organs will gradually break down, leading to the risk of premature death. Ageing is therefore an incredibly serious issue.

Chapter 3

The Magic Bullet to Youth: Anti-Ageing Hormones

THE NATURAL ASSUMPTION is that, if you see the error of your ways and consciously try to stop smoking, cut down on drinking, late nights and stress and look at your diet, your body will become better equipped to block out ageing. So far, so true, but there's one major missing link: although you will have taken action to prevent the bad habits that cause ageing, nothing whatsoever has been done to stop the ageing process itself, or even reverse the damage that it does to your body. So, how can you make your body young again? As well as adopting healthier habits, you need to block – and even reverse – ageing. This is the missing link and I'm about to reveal how to tackle the root cause of ageing so you can turn back the clock and look young again. With the Dr Nirdosh Anti-Ageing Plan, you'll live longer, look younger and have a sexier, younger body with the strength of a teenager and the libido to match!

To recapture your youth, you must stop the degeneration process and switch back to a body that regenerates itself to its younger state. So, how is this possible? The answer lies in our hormonal chemistry. Hormonal change is key to ageing, so read on to learn about a special, anti-ageing group of these chemical messengers.

THE YOUTH MESSENGERS

Special chemicals in the body (I call them the 'Youth Messengers') are really exciting because they have the skill to rebuild it. Until now I have only talked about the causes of ageing, but I have developed a way to take this a step further in allowing these hormones to slow down and even reverse the effects of ageing. When the body ages, this is simply caused by a failure in its ability to regenerate. Instead of enabling us to grow younger each day, we become older – in other words, the regeneration process stops and degeneration takes over. This is ageing, and our hormones play a large part in this process.

So, what are hormones? Hormones are tiny chemical messengers that travel around the body and tell it what to do. They keep us alive and in a balanced state, allowing the human body to function as one unit. Hormones tell the heart when to contract, they allow periods and pregnancy to occur, they determine our moods, run our immune system and control our metabolism and body weight; they allow us to eat food and digest it; also to think and they let our bodies grow. Most importantly, they encourage our body to regenerate and determine the rate at which we age.

If, for example, the body endures stress, then the 'stress hormone' cortisol is instantly released. Cortisol enters the body and sets in motion a 'flight or fight' reaction – an anxious, rushed state that enables us to handle any sudden dramatic instances that occur. In other words, the body releases stress hormones.

If you're about to go on one of those wild experiences such as swimming with sharks in a metal cage, the chances are you'll be feeling pretty scared. This fear signals to the body that you need help. The body reacts accordingly, and the chemicals inside undergo a sudden change. Stress floods your body with the hormone adrenaline, which allows you to deal with any sudden stress. Adrenaline causes your heartbeat to increase, blood pressure rises and you get a sudden burst of extra energy; now your muscles are ready for you to flee. The extra energy allows you to become that bit stronger than you would normally be.

What has just occurred is that the body's internal defence mechanism has kicked in to help you handle any situation. All this has been achieved through hormones. The mass rush of adrenaline causes your body to block out pain for a short period of time so you can complete your task without feeling any fear or aches, that's the power of hormones. In fact, hormones send signals to all parts of our body – organs, tissues and cells – so that we can perform tasks and make adjustments to adapt to any situation. Central to helping the body stay in good health, they work on a vast array of sections, including the digestive systems, sex organs and taste buds; they even determine how we age in our faces. Almost every component inside the body depends on hormones.

HOW HORMONES AGE US

During a lifetime, the human body experiences a massive change in hormonal activity. A younger body is naturally abundant in hormones, their sole purpose being to handle puberty. Once the body reaches puberty, the role of hormones changes as the body alters again and, at this stage, they aid us to successfully reach adulthood. As soon as we get there, it's all change again. Hormone levels diminish due to the everyday lifestyle choices we make and the consequence of this is progressive degeneration of the body or our old enemy: ageing.

Predominant factors such as smoking, alcohol, foods laden in fat and sugar, late nights, stress and static sedentary living, as well as the ageing process itself, all contribute to the changing role of hormones. If we continue to live a lifestyle dominated by these habits, eventually the impact will take its toll: the body becomes stressed and suddenly starts to release bad hormones, including one of the most dangerous of all: cortisol. As you have already learned, the stress hormone allows the body to adequately handle dramatic, high-anxiety states. However, there is a real problem here: the release of cortisol is meant to be a rare, short-term safety mechanism to occur only when needed. Long term, it is not good for the body, despite the fact that, in today's society, stressful experiences are a regular part of our daily routine.

When cortisol is released frequently and remains abundant in the system, it hampers the body's ability to stay young. Indeed, it takes over and starts to diminish the regeneration process, placing the body in a state of degeneration. When your body remains in this cortisol-releasing state, it is ageing. Prolonged

34

bouts of this negative cycle are responsible for your current health, body shape and facial structure.

As we age, the body changes and so too do our hormones. The hormones that once helped the body to grow stronger day by day are slowly taken over by the hormones that cause stress due to our hectic lifestyles and habits. Over time, the body becomes composed of more bad hormones than good ones and it's not just lifestyle, but ageing itself that causes the hormones to change. Collectively, the hormones necessary to maintain youth, virility and strength start to diminish; this in itself induces ageing.

Now you know that hormones can also cause negative as well as positive effects in the body. How you normally treat your body determines the hormones floating around inside you at any one time. If you don't look after yourself, then unhealthy, age-prone hormones will quickly replace the beneficial ones. Let's take a closer look at hormones, bad and good.

Bad Hormones

- Insulin – a storage hormone that drives glucose out of the blood and into cells, stabilising blood sugar levels. The brain receives glucose as energy fuel, while the liver and muscles store energy as glycogen. Insulin pushes lipids into adipocytes (fat cells) for storage, promoting weight gain.
- Cortisol – a stress hormone. Long-term release can cause insulin resistance, obesity, weakened immunity, skin collagen breakdown and digestion problems. Most importantly, it counteracts the good anti-ageing hormones.

- Adrenaline – also called epinephrine. Acts as both a hormone and a neurotransmitter. It acts on the nervous system and helps the body to engage in the 'fight or flight' reaction. With it comes the rising of blood pressure, dilation of pupils, availability of fatty acids and an increase of glucose in the blood. The nervous system becomes activated by stimulations of danger or thrill.

- Nora-adrenaline – has two prime functions. The first is as a stress hormone during the 'fight or flight' reaction (muscles are gorged with blood and both energy levels and heart rate are increased). Its other function is as a neurotransmitter and anti-inflammatory agent in the brain.

These are known collectively as the 'bad ageing hormones' because, in large, constant doses, they will have a negative effect on the body. In short bursts, yes, they can prove beneficial, but imagine a body composed of high amounts of insulin, cortisol and adrenaline. It would appear prematurely aged, overweight and the skin would appear dull and wrinkled. Internally, there would be low energy levels, possible heart problems, recurring infections and digestive problems.

Junk foods, too much caffeine, financial difficulties, work issues, the responsibilities of life, unsettling changes such as relationship break-ups and moving house all cause chemical imbalance in the body. This leads to concerns such as depression, muscular deterioration, loss of sex drive, lack of mobility, facial ageing in the form of wrinkly, sagging skin, plus medical complications such as high blood pressure, even strokes. The bad hormones combine to accelerate age damage.

Good Hormones

- Human Growth Hormone (HGH)
- Dehydroepiandrosterone (DHEA)
- Pregnenolone
- Melatonin
- Thyroid hormone
- Oestrogen
- Testosterone
- Progesterone
- Endorphins (a feel-good hormone that gives a natural high)

Conversely, the good hormones help the body to achieve growth and recovery. Once activated, they work to ensure your sexual functionality stays at peak performance, the body remains young through growth and repair, your face stays young, firm, plump and unlined, the body remains in good health through optimum organ health and you live longer. The problem is that, as we age, the good hormones disappear, in fact, so much so that, by the time you reach 40, you may have lost 50 per cent of the magical anti-ageing Growth Hormone that you had in your teen years. Fast forward and by the time you reach your 60th birthday, just 20 years later, you could have lost a massive 80 per cent of the Growth Hormone that you had in your youth.

Chapter 4

The Revelation Unveiled

HORMONES FASCINATED ME while at medical school and so I researched further into their workings and possibilities; I also wanted to learn how good hormones slowly evaporate and are overtaken by bad hormones with age. So, why does this happen?

I discovered that, when catabolism (molecular breakdown) – or body degeneration – occurs, it takes place faster than anabolism (molecular synthesis) – or regeneration – as we start to age. This means that degeneration is in fact more rapid than repair, so the body ages. What I noticed was that stress hormones generally cause catabolism, whereas good hormones create anabolism.

I realised that, if we could only prevent break down and reprogramme the body to remain in an anabolic regeneration state, then ageing might be defied. What happens if we starve the ageing body of the resources it needs to recreate youth and restore the original powers of its teens? If this could be achieved, then the effects of ageing would be undone: you would look young, your face would once more be wrinkle-free, your body redefined, your sex drive would never die and you would live longer.

AGEING THE NIRDOSH WAY

Let me reveal to you the revolutionary Dr Nirdosh way to tackle ageing: through the power of hormones, the body can become younger and resist the ageing process. After a decade of intense medical research, I devised a unique way to activate and naturally reinject anti-ageing hormones within the body by means of stimulation from Growth Hormone boosters.

The Dr Nirdosh Anti-Ageing Plan comprises naturally safe, non-surgical and non-invasive mechanisms using the body's own anti-ageing chemicals to rush youth back into the system so you look younger and sexier for longer. This miracle scheme floods important anti-ageing hormones into the system to put an out-of-control, ageing body back in control of itself. In just six weeks, it helps to reverse the ageing process and recaptures youth.

Many clients who follow my anti-ageing plan have embraced it as an ongoing life solution, rather than a short-term miracle fix. They incorporate it into their everyday routine and love it because the Dr Nirdosh anti-ageing lifestyle makes you look hot! It's a way to ensure your body remains in tip-top condition so that it performs at peak levels. You'll look and feel decades younger, enjoy heightened sexual feelings and have bounds of energy and confidence.

The special Nirdosh effect removes the body from a degenerative, ageing state and places it in a regenerative, anti-ageing state; it will steer you away from the catabolic breakdown that leads to facial drooping, muscle loss and general daily ageing. Instead, your body enters an anabolic state, protected from bone demineralisation, muscle tissue evaporation, skin thinning, weight gain and a low sex drive. The new anabolic state entered by your body allows it to heal and repair itself from within.

Ageing is both internal and external. However, it mainly starts from within and that's why it's so vital that we reverse the internal damage that creates the snowball effect of wear and tear in the first place. Stopping the internal damage processes allows your body to switch into heal-and-replenish mode – which is where we all need to be – to allow the body to de-age naturally.

My discovery that anti-ageing hormones hold the secret to eternal youth laid the foundations for the four-step life plan, which makes it possible to reignite declining levels of youth chemicals. The plan reshapes the physique and boosts the health of the inner organs, while helping to enliven skin-cell immunity. This whole process allows both face and body to win the fight against ageing.

PRESCRIPTION FOR A YOUNGER FACE AND SEXIER BODY

As already stated, the Dr Nirdosh anti-ageing discipline is a unique four-step combination of the following: exercise techniques, a diet plan, supplements and skincare treatments. Carrying out these steps together, we are going to stimulate endogenous synthesis of anti-ageing hormones and boost skin-cell immunity (i.e. the inner body production of anti-ageing hormones as opposed to those taken from external sources such as injections).

Internally and externally, the four-step clinical effect opposes the ageing process, recapturing youth, inside and out. It will put decades of lost youth back into your system.

ANTI-AGEING HORMONE-BOOSTING EXERCISES

My short and unique way of exercising amplifies secretion of anti-ageing hormones, especially Human Growth Hormone (HGH), and prevents the catabolic breakdown that occurs when you work out the wrong way.

Specialised techniques force your muscular system to reach maximum activation levels, flooding anti-ageing hormones into the body and rebuilding lean tissue fibres so that an all-over firming, lifting effect occurs. This exercise plan helps combat sarcopenia (the age-related loss of essential muscle tissue), stimulates lipolysis (fat burning), balances the ratio of body fat to muscle, makes organs healthier, enhances the libido, strengthens immunity and tightens the skin. The result is a trimmer, sexier body and a firmer face.

THE ANTI-AGEING DIET

This is a specialist diet consisting of three structured meals per day with six-hour fasting periods in between. Each meal contains a bounty of potent high-quality nutrients and the amino acids that help boost production of Human Growth Hormone (HGH). A diet containing the amino acids arginine, glutamine, ornithine and glycine helps put the body on track to manufacture skin collagen and anti-ageing hormones by encouraging it to produce HGH and helping to power collagen synthesis.

The Dr Nirdosh Plan including food fuelled with nourishing nutrients, combined with the six-hour fasting phases, helps slow down the ageing process and turns on your longevity gene so you look younger. It also promotes weight loss and increases your life span. Protein synthesis is increased, cell life extended and the production of free radicals minimised. (Free radicals are unstable molecules that have lost part of their structure and are looking to steal the missing part from a nearby, complete molecule. This molecule would then be rendered unstable and would be on the prowl to steal from another. It's like a chain reaction that goes on until you feed it the missing component in the form of an antioxidant.) My eating plan helps to overcome premature apoptosis (early cell death), a detrimental reaction in which speedy cell damage means cells are lost faster than they can be repaired and replaced. Eat in this way and you will look younger for longer!

SKIN AND BODY DE-AGEING SUPPLEMENTS

With age, the skin – like the rest of the body – gradually loses the ability to heal deep wrinkles. These skin wounds begin in the innermost layer of the skin (the dermis) and a surgeon's knife cannot change the ageing rate of it. This dermal layer contains skin collagen – supportive fibres responsible for maintaining facial firmness and plumpness.

My supplement plan provides the body with the anti-ageing nutrients so easily missed, putting the absent components into a metabolic process so the body works like a newly serviced engine. Strengthened inner immunity helps the body fight infection and ageing diseases, while providing skin cells with the correct healing elements to add rigour to skin-cell immunity so the scars of ageing – wrinkles – can be repaired. The Dr Nirdosh supplement concept helps make the skin and body immune to ageing, giving you the best skin possible and a body roaring with health.

SKIN DEFENCE AND RENEWAL

Using dedicated anti-wrinkle ingredients, my skincare programme treats damage according to age, gender and skin type. It provides a defence plan to ensure skin surfaces are properly equipped to combat environmental ageing through targeted topical preparations that guard the outer skin surface.

The anti-ageing support works to reduce facial wrinkles, fine lines, rebalance skin pores, reduce pigmentation and age spots, improve texture and prevent acne from flaring up.

Read on to discover more about my anti-ageing secrets and how to gain a younger-looking, flawless complexion just as you become older.

Chapter 5

The Dr Nirdosh Anti-Ageing Body Plan

IN JUST SIX weeks, I can change the way your body looks forever. You will learn to look younger, lose fat, regain muscle tissue, strengthen skin collagen and fix a damaged, out-of-shape body by harnessing your own natural anti-ageing hormones.

The key is Exercise Induced Growth Hormone Release (EIGR), a foolproof system for men and women that works on specific muscle groups and forces the body to regenerate. It's a far cry from traditional methods, which lead to the majority of us exercising completely wrongly and almost certainly damaging our bodies daily by following the instructions of personal trainers and gym regimes.

Jogging and other cardiovascular exercise carried out for periods of 30–40 minutes at a time can cause severe signs of ageing, forcing muscle breakdown and blocking the major anti-ageing Growth Hormone. Under my plan, each session lasts just 20 minutes a day, fitting easily into your lifestyle. Unique movements will open up gateways in your body and persuade the hypothalamic-pituitary system in the brain to pour out powerful anti-ageing hormones. (The hypothalamus and pituitary are both small glands located in the brain that work together to control the release of certain hormones including growth hormone.) These include the bodily superpower Human Growth Hormone, a magical youth booster and a favourite of celebrities. The stars will try anything to keep these chemicals stacked in their body, as they know they can make a 50-year-old look and act like someone in their twenties.

These anti-ageing chemicals will remain secreted in your body for 24–48 hours after your workout. They do amazing things to help thicken and firm facial skin, rebalance the body-tissue composition of muscle to fat, improve your overall wellbeing and encourage beauty and youth. That's why the Dr Nirdosh Plan is the celebrity favourite workout – one that until now has been kept under wraps.

Once you have finished working out, you'll have a body brimming with the chemicals that help block ageing and work hard to make it look young again. It's amazing to think that you can achieve all this in just 20 minutes each day but this is no ordinary exercise plan – it is the only one that defies ageing. In that golden 20 minutes, the body will repair and even reverse age damage so you look sexier and more youthful.

THE TIMEFRAME

You will exercise for three days on and then take one day off – so, if you work out on Monday, Tuesday and Wednesday, you will have Thursday off for your body to recover. The day off is known as the '3R', which stands for repair + refuel + reverse ageing. The 3R day will:

- **Repair** the muscle fibres that have just been stimulated by the workouts so they become stronger and firmer and induce regeneration of the skin.
- **Refuel** the body with vital anti-ageing nutrients (including amino acids to make proteins), Growth Hormone boosters, vitamins, antioxidants and minerals to enhance age defences.
- **Reverse ageing** by changing the body composition to a well-proportioned muscle-to-fat ratio, diminishing wrinkles and repairing age damage, while flooding your system with anti-ageing hormones.

If you skip 3R, you will be physically and mentally strained and unable to continue. This leads to burnout, resulting in failure. It's easy to get addicted to the plan and miss 3R. If you do, you'll need to take 10 steps back and start all over again.

You may work out in the day or evening, the choice is yours, but make sure you exercise at least two hours after your meal. Actually, evening workouts are best done before a meal; similarly, morning workouts are best pre-breakfast.

You want your liver glycogen stores to become as depleted as possible so your body turns to fat for energy. Studies have shown that working out on a fasted, empty stomach causes fat burning to rocket. That's why morning times are great – you've just fasted overnight for at least eight hours. On this plan, your body also continues to bolster fat loss for hours after the workouts.

As you will be developing more muscle tissue (which is highly active metabolically), your body will use up more calories, even at rest. Every angle of the new you will be redesigned to shed more fat and stay lean.

If possible, start before breakfast when your fat-burning mechanisms are most active and your carbohydrate levels have depleted. The morning allows the body to use fat as the primary fuel source during your workout. Great, so not only are you going to look younger, but you'll also lose fat right from your first session.

But the plan is not confined to mornings, it is flexible. Whichever time you choose to work out, be consistent: if you train in the early evening, try to stick to this time, and likewise with mornings. That way your body will adjust more easily to your new lifestyle.

SIX WEEKS TO A NEW YOU

Exercise for 20 minutes each day without any days off except for the 3R rest day. In this way, you will be targeting redevelopment and growth, and this will be achieved with astonishing results over a short period of time.

As your body emerges looking more youthful, not only will you dramatically alter your physique but you'll also encourage advanced cellular immunity and DNA protection so you can live a longer, healthier life.

WHY MUSCLE?

Muscle tissue stores glutamine, the most abundant of the amino acids, which are the building blocks of life in the body, and a serious elevator of Human Growth Hormone (HGH).

Ideally, we do not want to lose any of our vital muscle tissue. If this decreases, levels of anti-ageing hormones diminish and the overlying skin has no support network beneath it, so the face sags and the body becomes flabby. When we lose muscle, we allow our bodies to rapidly become tarnished by ageing. Lose muscle and you lose youth.

How the Dr Nirdosh Muscle Sets Aid Youth

The special Dr Nirdosh method has been meticulously devised to reconfigure your internal body structure so you shrug off evidence of ageing while performing the exercises. The miracle science that makes this all possible is fast-twitch fibres in the muscles themselves.

Muscle is made up of two types of fibre: slow-twitch fibres (Type 1) and fast-twitch fibres (Type 2). With age, the Type 2 fibres can quickly die: a dormant body that doesn't use muscle on a daily basis soon progresses to age-related loss of muscle, which seriously hampers our quality of life and is also a sign of ageing. These are the fibres of youth and a major factor in turning back the age clock as they help release anti-ageing Growth Hormone.

We are going to reactivate them and promote muscle regrowth, a process that enhances production of these key fibres. My workout will boost facial-muscle firmness, perk up your bum, tighten the hips, narrow the waist and cause the body to rid itself of fat, while bolstering the activity of anti-ageing hormones.

Finally, you should write down how you're looking, how you feel and how much you have changed. This is vital because you will start to change shape and look different after just one week and the realisation that you are changing will encourage you to continue. If you should ever stop the plan, go right back and read through your notes to see what stage you reached so you remember how effective it is. This will motivate you to jump back aboard quickly!

THE MOVEMENTS

The exercises are divided into two sections: upper and lower body.

On the first day you will be working the upper body, the next day the lower body and then back to the upper body on the third day before moving on to 3R on the fourth day. After the rest day, you return to the plan and begin with the lower body, followed by the upper body the day after, then the lower and so on in a continual rotation. For the first 20 minutes of your first day, you'll be working the upper regional muscle groups: the back, shoulders, chest, biceps and triceps. The plan activates the upper-body muscle groups through the whole workout.

Using your muscles will rectify the damage of muscle-tissue loss and counteract sarcopenia, a progressive, serious medical condition of age-related muscular breakdown that leads to sagginess, loss of power and a decline in mobility. Plus, it stimulates the hypothalamic-pituitary system in the brain to boost the release of Growth Hormone Releasing Hormone (GHRH). This then attaches to receptors in the pituitary gland, also located in the brain and the treasure chest that holds Growth Hormone, which will be discharged into the blood to be transported to your organs so your face and body look younger. This completes Day One.

On Day Two, you will be working the lower-body parts and muscle groups including the front thighs (quadriceps) and the backs of the legs (hamstrings), the bum (gluteus) and the calves (gastrocnemius and soleus), as well as the stomach (abdominals). Again, the plan is performed via resistance movements to transform the shape of your lower body, while placing it in an anti-ageing state.

Return to the upper-body exercises above on Day Three.

THE TWO-SET PRINCIPLE

You will be doing supersets: two sets carried out one after the other without any rest in between. One set uses a heavy weight with low repetitions, while the next is a light set with high repetitions. In this way you not only target the muscle group, but also specifically stimulate fast-twitch muscle fibres.

On the first set, you must choose a weight that you feel will test you. It cannot be too light or the right muscle fibres won't get working, but it must not be too heavy either or you won't be able to perform the movement correctly.

You should only be able to do 8–10 repetitions – no less and certainly no more! With the weight you have chosen, the last 2–3 reps should feel quite demanding. If it's too easy, then you're not engaging those fast-twitch fibres; too heavy and you risk injury.

After you've completed your first set comfortably and finished the first 8–10 reps, start your second set immediately. Now get ready to work the same muscle group and fibres again. This time you do this without a pause and no weights, or you can pick up a dramatically lighter weight because you'll be doing more repetitions.

On the second set, do 15–20 faster, powered reps, but make sure your weight is not too heavy or you won't reach the required number. That's why it's a good idea to perform the second set with just the bar and no weights added, or very light ones to begin with. Use faster, more explosive movements. Remember, you want to see that face- and body-lift! Once you've finished your second set, you have performed your first superset and completed your first muscle group exercise, which has activated your fast-twitch muscle fibres to help maximise Growth Hormone secretion.

So let's recap: you do two sets of reps to make one superset. They are:

- **Set One:** 8–10 reps with fairly heavy weights and slow controlled movements.
- **Set Two:** 15–20 reps with light weights and fast explosive movements.

Both sets are carried out continuously without a rest in between. Really, the only time you stop is to switch the weights. Once you have done this, you have completed a superset.

For women, a good starting point for upper-body workout heavy weights would be dumbbells of 2–3kg, followed by lighter dumbbells of 0.5–1kg. For the lower-body legs workout, a starting weight for the heavy set could again be around 2–3 kg and the lighter set should begin with no weights at all as leg exercises are more difficult to do than upper body exercises as the body itself already has a weight-bearing effect. Men should be able to do double the weight recommended for women.

To gauge whether a weight is heavy enough for the first set of 8–10 reps, perform one of the exercises with it. If you get to 10 too easily, the weight is too light; if you struggle, shake and barely reach 8, then the weight is too heavy. Use the same test for the lighter set.

For these exercises, good form is key – never compromise technique for weight. The movements are precise and it's easy to remove the load from the muscle you are meant to be working on. Focus on the muscle you are working, feel it contract and relax again and make sure your weight really works it.

Upper Body

We only ever do one superset for each body part. This works the selected muscle group and the fast-twitch fibres of that muscle group. For example, once you have completed your superset on the chest, rest for one minute before moving on to the next muscle group, your shoulders, and perform a superset on them.

Now take a breather for between 30 seconds and 1 minute before you move on to the next body part and muscle group. This allows you to regain your energy and breath to go again. It also keeps your heart rate elevated and the muscle fibres engorged with nutrient-rich blood, sending amplified signals to the brain to release anti-ageing hormones.

Don't worry if you feel slightly out of breath: this workout also doubles up as your correct cardiovascular exercise programme and will strengthen your heart and encourage your body to become a fat-burning machine. Awesome!

Now move on to the next muscle group, doing a weighted set

of 8–10 reps, followed by a non-weighted set of 15–20. The Dr Nirdosh system of supersets really gets to the core of the fast-twitch fibres and stimulates hundreds of muscle-nerve motor units, exploiting EIGR.

In the first, heavy part of the double sets, you must control the weights and ensure you lower them slowly into position. Really squeeze those muscles at the extreme contraction of the movement, so the push is a clean, swift, powerful movement, taking the weight to its starting position.

Do the second, lighter set relatively fast so it resembles a sprinting motion.

The plan requires you to do five supersets in every upper-body session so you work the chest, shoulders, back, biceps and triceps.

Lower Body

Your second-day workout covers the lower body, exercising the fronts and backs of the legs, the calves, the bum and the abdominals.

Note that on the lower body you will also be working five muscle groups. Compared to the upper body, the lower body needs more precision to anti-age, so really focus on good form. The session is still 20 minutes and again you must perform a superset: one set slowly with heavy weights and low reps, the other fast with light weights and high reps on each muscle group.

As before, in each first set, you must control the weights and really squeeze at the peak of the contraction phase, then return to the starting position with a clean, swift motion. Remember, the second set of the superset is a fast, explosive movement.

So now you will have completed the upper body on Day One and the lower body on Day Two. Using supersets you have done four special things:

Reintroduced the fast-twitch muscle fibres that normally wither away with age. The anaerobic (without oxygen) working of these fibres helps elevate youth in each superset by producing an environment of lactate, nitric oxide, nerve stimulation, change in acid-base balance and catecholamines. These can mega-elevate Growth Hormone within the body. This action is best achieved when high-intensity, high-weight-load exercises are performed for specific periods. Studies have shown that, when lactate levels are above the threshold for more than 10 minutes, these are potent Growth Hormone releasers. My plan will take you way above the lactate threshold, significantly amplifying anti-ageing hormones.

This routine also doubles as the correct cardiovascular session because it safely raises your resting heart rate and eliminates fat by boosting thermogenic fat-burning mechanisms (i.e. the rise in metabolism caused by the creation of heat energy in the body, promoting weight loss and fat burning) while you are working out and for hours afterwards. In addition, it helps to improve the muscularity of the heart, so strengthening the cardiovascular system. Even after you have finished your exercises, the hormones that have flooded your body can be enhanced for up to 48 hours after a session so your body continues, round the clock, to fend off ageing. If you really want to kick-start your metabolism, try drinking green tea with lemon before you work out.

These exercises make you look sexy and ageless: a knifeless, tighten-and-lift effect will occur naturally as you increase your body resilience and muscle mass. Facial-muscle firmness is boosted through the upper-body exercises, and you'll also get a rounder, perkier bum that will seriously turn a few heads! Your hips will tighten, you'll lose those fatty love handles and your waist will start to shrink away as you become thinner and leaner. Once your body starts to shed fat, this will be replaced with a sexier and more shapely, defined frame so you look younger, tighter and healthier.

Upper-Body Muscles

The chest muscle (pectoralis) is a major muscle group and will be the first muscle worked on your upper body. You will be required to perform a superset to stimulate the chest pectorals. This routine is great because it lifts the whole breast and chest section. Aged saggy breasts benefit immensely here as the chest region becomes firmer and you will experience a natural boob-lift. For men, this is a serious part of your plan – you'll start to develop model-like pectorals and turn a flabby chest section to a neat size and more defined shape.

As the fat begins to shrink, the sexy chest muscles hidden underneath it will start to be revealed. Currently, you may have fatty deposits and overlying, saggy skin but this will not be the case once you join the plan: as fat levels drop, the fruits of your efforts begin to show.

These exercises work on the shoulders (the deltoid muscles) to give you a sexy V-shape frame and counteract narrowed shoulders that may have dwindled with age. They will also tighten facial muscles, firming the jowls. Your front and back shoulders too will become rounded and well defined. This routine also tackles a major ageing concern: turkey neck. As you progress further into the plan you will feel your skin start to tighten under the neck and around the jaw line so saggy neck skin becomes firmer and more structured-looking.

Many of you may have noticed that you have excess loose fat on your back that rolls over on itself, especially at the sides near the underarms. With women, this is a major problem. When you wear a bra, your back fat falls over it and looks unattractive; it also feels uncomfortable. The back is a major muscle group (latissimus dorsi) on the plan, which will give you a significant improvement.

As you lose the fat, your sleek and sexy new back without the rolls will unveil itself. The plan allows both men and women to eliminate a bent middle-aged back and create a well-postured one in its place without accumulating fat to mask its shape.

Bingo wings (or extra fat and no muscle support under your arms) are also a problem for men and women. Working your triceps will help you to quickly lose the saggy, fatty tissue and tone up flaccid arm muscles.

Bicep movements will give you shapely arms and eradicate the wobbly skin that occurs with age. This is a problem for both women and men as this is a place where fat accumulates, muscle tissue is soon lost and the arms quickly become lumpy and loose; it stops many people from wearing short tops in the summer and can create a loss of confidence.

Your bicep routines will change all this: they will give you hot, shapely and tight biceps. Initially, they will be hidden under the fat, like other muscles around the body, but, as soon as it starts to vanish, you'll get gorgeous arms that you will love showing off. Your confidence will go through the roof as your arms become stronger.

Lower-Body Muscles

'Spare tyre syndrome' is the name for those extra rolls of fat around the stomach due to mid-abdominal weight gain. Finally, you can rid yourself of those horrid fat rolls and create a slimmer, more defined abdominal region in the process. So, why is this important? If you do not work your stomach muscles and only lose the fat, then you will have layers of excess skin that you will not be able to lose or tighten because, although you will have shed the fat, you will have no muscle to show. The result is surplus, sagging skin that you will hate forever. With the exercises, you will lose the fat and your new abdominal muscles will start to come through so everyone can see the result of your efforts.

Thighs have a tendency to hoard fat and can become lumpy and wobbly. My leg workouts will help to tighten slack skin and firm underlying muscle. The front thigh region becomes more beautifully shaped, trimmer and elongated.

When it comes to the legs, a lot of women make the mistake of thinking that dieting or loads of cardio exercises will do the trick, but, if you have no muscle prominence on the thighs and lose just the fat, then you'll be left with scrawny pins. Well-developed muscle tissue in the legs gives them a curvaceous, eye-catching look.

The plan also deals with one of the biggest concerns for women's legs: cellulite. Due to the higher concentration of oestrogen and progesterone in women, the female body is genetically programmed to house more fat than muscle compared to a man's body, which carries more testosterone, an anti-ageing hormone that enhances muscle composition and vigour. Supersets on the back thighs will work the hamstring back-thigh muscles. Through fast-paced workouts, you will also eliminate the fat and cellulite on the back of the legs, while defining muscle. This is like a natural liposuction treatment but better because it kick-starts the shift of adipocytes (fat cells) and lipolysis and actually breaks them down. My routine produces more slender, gorgeously shapely sexy legs in women, while men will have more muscular and defined legs with greater power and muscle mass.

As they age, most women experience a saggy bum that has lost the battle with gravity and is falling southwards. For some, it is so bad that it's hard to see where the legs end and the buttocks start, as they seem to have merged. This happens when you lose the muscle tissue that holds your buttocks up. The supersets target this region directly so you can regain the perfect, peachy derrière. Over the next six weeks, you'll learn to love your behind again and enjoy your sexy curves!

Our calves hold the weight of the legs and help us walk. They need to be youthful and strong to ensure that the legs can carry this load without problems. My plan will reshape them and give a more striking contour, while enhancing their power.

Remember, once you begin to lose the layers of fatty tissue, your body will be sexier and tighter. If you simply lose the weight and you do not have muscle in its place, then you will reveal only a bony, aged and haggard look.

LET'S START WORKING OUT
Upper-Body Workout

We'll begin with some stretching. Wear comfortable, loose clothing suitable for indoor exercises using weights. If you go to a gym or fitness club, then you should find the Anti-Ageing Body Plan a breeze as the resistance machines, free weights and a basic weights bench will all be there. Otherwise, you will need to buy a basic set of dumbbells with pairs of 0.5–1kg, 2–3kg and 4–5kg weights. If you are exercising at home, you will also have to buy a basic weights bench on which the back can be raised and flattened. Whether exercising at home or at the gym, you will need a stopwatch to time your exercises.

To minimise the risk of injury or pulling a muscle, first stretch your arms up towards the ceiling. Hold for 10 seconds and then bring them down.

With palms facing upwards, stretch your arms out at each side as far as they will go. Hold for 10 seconds and relax again.

Now, with your left hand, reach down over your head to touch your back as far as your hand will go. Hold for 10 seconds and then relax. Repeat with the right.

Bend your left leg at the knee so your left foot reaches towards your left buttock. Use your left hand to grip your foot and hold for 10 seconds. You should feel the stretch in your quadriceps, the muscles at the top of the legs. **Do not bounce the movements and only stretch as far as you can sensibly go. Never force a stretch as this can cause injury.** Now relax and then do the same for the other leg.

Finally, gradually curl your body over to reach towards your toes, bending your back. Hold this for 10 seconds and then relax.

You are now ready to begin the workout itself. **If you decide to skip the stretching process, your Anti-Ageing Plan will be brought to a standstill and you risk injury.** On the first day, we will work the upper body together. With just 20 minutes, we need to get straight down to it.

To do this, you need a bottle of water, the stopwatch, free weights or resistance machines and a flat surface, such as a bench. **Water is essential: you must stay hydrated throughout the session so sip water during the breaks specified. Avoid sugary drinks – you don't want glucose rushes to play havoc with your blood-sugar levels.**

Never have more than a 1-minute break. This is, after all, a cardiovascular session too, which raises your resting heart rate so it's important not to go over the allocated time.

Step 1: Dumbbell Press

The first superset will work the chest. Choose a set of dumbbells which you feel you can comfortably do 8–10 reps with. Now start the stopwatch, grab the weights and lie down on the weights bench.

You are going to do an exercise called the Dumbbell Press. Hold the weights directly above your head. Breathe in deeply and slowly lower to each side of your chest so you almost touch the outer part of the chest. Hold for one second. Now slowly, and with control, exhale and breathe out as you lift the weights up again to return to your starting position and complete one rep. Repeat for rep two and continue until you have completed 8–10 reps, then place your weights on the floor.

61

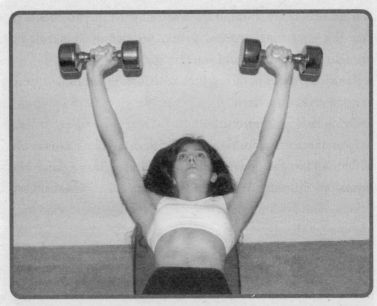

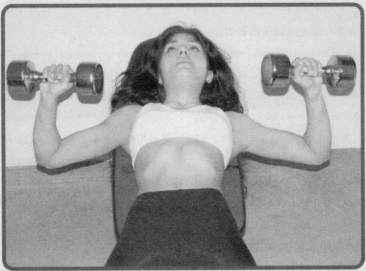

The Dumbbell Press

Immediately, without rest, grab some lighter weights. You will now do a fast set of 15–20 reps, so make sure the weight is not too heavy for you. Return to the starting position on the bench. This time not only will you increase the repetition range to 15–20, but you must also do faster, more explosive moves, while always ensuring they are controlled.

From the starting position (see photo opposite), first lower the weights all the way down to the outer chest regions again while breathing in deeply. When you reach the level of your chest, breathe out to take the weight back up again in a fast, explosive movement without pause.

From the starting position again, immediately bring the weight back down towards the chest and then back to the top to make 2 reps. Continue for 15–20 reps. **The reps should be carried out with speed and control and without pause. Always ensure that you breathe in as you lower the weight and out as you push up.**

Once you have completed this, take a look at your stopwatch. Note the time without stopping (it should be between 1 minute 30 seconds and 2 minutes). You have just blasted your first superset. Now take a breather for 30 seconds to 1 minute – you deserve it!

Step 2: Shoulder Superset
Move straight on to the Shoulder Superset, this time using the shoulder dumbbell press. Raise the back of the bench so that you are sitting upright with your back supported, grab a set of the heavier weights and get ready for the first part of the exercise: the slow, controlled movement of 8–10 reps.

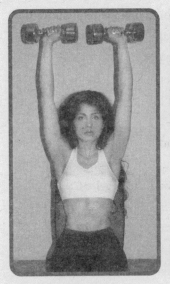 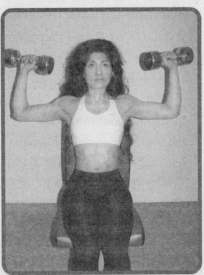

Shoulder Superset

Slowly take the weights down close to your shoulders, breathing in as they are lowered. Hold for 1 second and then return to the starting position using a clean, swift swiping movement to complete one rep. Repeat for rep number two, but make sure you breathe correctly. Now do 8–10 reps of the shoulder press.

Immediately you will feel the heat burning in your shoulders. It's great because this is lactic acid which tells us that the muscles are working and it's also the signal for Growth Hormone secretion to start: EIGR is occurring!

Now change to the lighter weights and get ready to blast out 15–20 reps. Remember not to pause this time, just get the reps out fast. Once you have finished, put the weights down. The Shoulder Superset is complete.

Take a look at your stopwatch. By now you should be between 4.5 minutes and 5 minutes into the plan. Note the time. Again, take a break of between 30 seconds and 1 minute. You're doing great!

Step 3: Back Rows

Break over. Get ready to blast the back with a superset exercise called Back Rows. You will be doing a rowing motion and this may feel awkward at the start, but you'll soon get used to it.

First, place one knee on the bench and your other leg on the floor, as shown. Lower your arm to the starting position (see over) and then lift the weight up, working your back shoulder blade and breathing in as you do so. Hold and then slowly return to the starting position, breathing out. When doing this movement, make sure you look ahead, not down.

The difference here is that the force is used in the pulling motion, whereas with the chest and shoulder movements the force is required in the pushing motion. Both require the same amount of effort and still work the fast-twitch muscle fibres. This time we will perform all the reps first in a slow controlled set and then a fast, explosive set, before moving on to work the other arm.

The concept of having no break between sets and intensely working one arm at a time activates fast-twitch fibres and encourages maximum Growth Hormone release. So, first do 8–10 reps with your right arm. As soon as you have done the required number of reps, put the weight down and immediately change to the lighter one. Without a pause, go

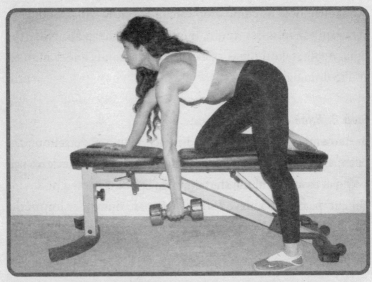

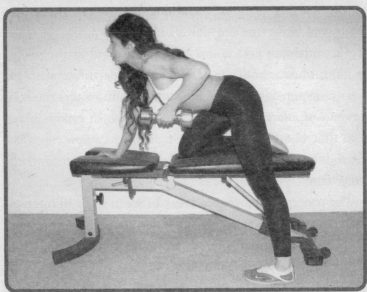

Back Rows

again with the same right arm and perform 15–20 reps. Remember, this time the explosive, fast and controlled movement is in the initial pulling motion. Go to the starting position and pull the weight up fast. Then, without a pause, move your arm straight down to do 2 reps. Continue until you have completed the set amount.

Remember, keep looking directly ahead throughout the exercise – this is the correct way to maximise the back muscle being activated and not the rest of your body, while also saving the neck from injury. Make sure you don't do any jerky movements with your neck and head – no up and down or side to side, and don't look up too far towards the ceiling.

Once you have completed 15–20 reps with your right arm, change the weight to your left arm and start again. First, do 8–10 reps with a heavy weight and then immediately change to the lighter weights and do 15–20 reps with the same arm.

Great, you have just finished your Back Superset. Now let's do a time check: you should have been working out for 7.5–8 minutes. Again, take a breather for 30 seconds to 1 minute.

Step 4: Biceps Dumbbell Curl

Let's move on to the arms. First, we'll do the biceps superset – a favourite of many people because working the biceps gives rapid results and you can see the change quite quickly.

A quick reminder: you're already halfway through your workout and the clock should be at about 10 minutes or so. You're almost done, so let's go! Grab a set of weights suitable for the first part of your bicep superset – 8–10 reps.

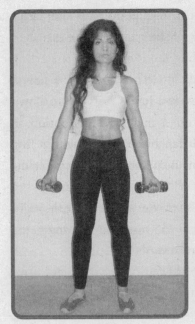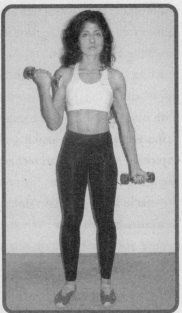

Bicep Dumbbell Curl

This exercise is called the Biceps Dumbbell Curl. Stand with your feet slightly apart, holding the dumbbells, as shown. This time we will rotate the movement. First, one rep with your left hand: bring it right up and curl the arm, breathing in slowly as you do so. Then take it back to the starting position, straight down by the sides of your hips and exhale at the same time. Now alternate to the right arm: bring the dumbbell up, while breathing in. Hold for 1 second and then bring it back down to the starting position, exhaling as you go. This counts as one rep.

Do the second rep: first the left curl, then the right to make 2 reps. Continue until you have completed 8–10 reps with each arm (total count should be 16–20 reps as you are alternating arms). Watch your biceps working as you complete the exercise – you'll see instant gains.

Change weights and go for the lighter option now, ready to do 15–20 reps. This time, when you bring the weights down with one arm, the other comes up in an alternating motion, so bring the weight up using your left bicep muscle with a fast, explosive, controlled movement. Remember to squeeze at the top of the contraction.

Now lower the weight and, as you do so, bring up the right arm at the same time. When your left dumbbell is down, the right one is all the way up. Lower the right straight away and, as you do so, lift your left arm to contract the left bicep, while the right bicep extends and relaxes. This swift, alternating motion is the way we do the fast part of the biceps superset. Keep a count of each rep and make sure each arm does 15–20 (the total count should reach 30–40 as you are alternating arms).

Make sure that you control your breathing, as described. Look at your biceps in a mirror as they contract and relax. This will help you to perfect the movement when you see your muscles working and feel the fast-twitch fibres stretching and contracting inside.

As soon as you finish, it's time to check your stopwatch: it must be between 10.5 and 11 minutes. Take a 1-minute breather and drink some water to keep you cool. If you're sweating, that's great – you have boosted your metabolism and you're burning fat. Your session is working and you have only two supersets left.

Step 5: Triceps Kickbacks

The next movement is called the Triceps Kickbacks, using one arm at a time in a similar movement to the way we worked the back and biceps. This will tighten the triceps muscles at the backs of your arms and get rid of those bingo wings.

This time perform all the reps with your right arm first before moving on to the left arm – there are no alternating movements. Kneel on a bench, as shown opposite. Begin with the right triceps: extend the arm back fully, hold for 1 second and then return to the starting position.

Remember to hold the position for 1 second before you bring your arm back to the starting position so the triceps muscle contracts (or shortens). You will feel the triceps working and soon see the results of the tighter skin and firmer muscles. Perform 8–10 reps with the right arm.

Once you have finished your set, change to the lighter weight and with the same arm, do 15–20 reps. Regulate your breathing to ensure you are not left gasping for breath.

Once you have completed the first arm, change to the second. Perform 8–10 weighted reps and then 15–20 lightweight ones. Be sure the second set of reps are fast-paced, controlled movements as you push backwards and out.

Immediately bring the weight down back to the starting point. Once you have done 15–20 reps, you will have completed your triceps superset. Do a time check: you should be at 14.5–15 minutes. Take a breather of between 30 seconds to 1 minute, and drink some more water to rehydrate. Almost done!

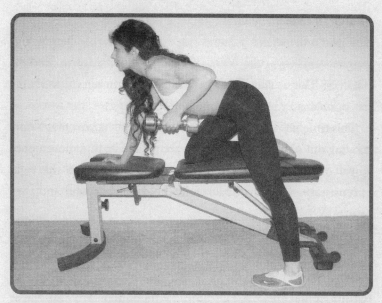

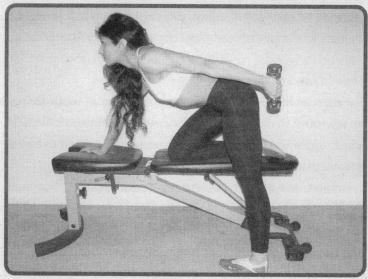

Triceps Kickbacks

Stretch to Finish

Now you must stretch again as you did at the start to loosen your muscles and lessen the onset of Delayed Onset Muscle Soreness (DOMS). This usually kicks in a day later but you can minimise the risk dramatically by doing your stretching exercises after workouts.

Once you have completed your stretches, look at your stopwatch. You have hit 20 minutes. Good job! You should be proud of yourself as you have just worked your muscles and fast-twitch fibres to optimise Human Growth Hormone (HGH) secretion.

Lower-Body Workout

As before, do some stretching to begin. Here, we have five supersets to work the fronts and backs of the legs, the bum, the calves and the abdominal muscles. This time, the movements will take a little longer so let's get started. Again, you need a stopwatch so you can keep track of your time and plenty of water to stay hydrated.

Step 1: The Squat

The muscles in the fronts of the legs are known as the quads and we are about to do a quad superset with a movement called The Squat, which is the most effective front-leg exercise. Grab a set of weights that will allow you to do a comfortable 8–10 reps.

Get into the starting position, as shown opposite. Now with the weights at your sides and your feet about shoulder width apart, toes slightly pointed outwards, lower yourself into the squat position, bending your knees until your thighs are parallel to the floor, as shown. Hold it there for 1 second and then raise yourself back to the starting position.

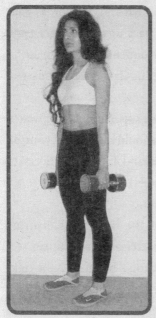 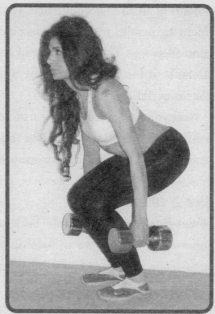

The Squat

Keep your back straight through The Squat and don't bend or curve it. That is one complete rep. **Remember to breathe in as you go down and exhale as you come up during your squat.** You will instantly feel the skin around the legs tighten and the muscles being awakened.

Holding the dumbbell weights at your sides again, complete another rep. Come down to the squat position. Hold for a second, and then go back up. This is 2 reps. Do 8–10 reps altogether.

Once you have completed your set, put the weights on the floor and now do a fast, explosive set of 15–20 reps with no weights at all and without pause. Go down and, as soon as your thighs are parallel with the floor, come back up again in a fast and controlled way. This is a powerful movement that uses a lot of strength so you do not need any weights in the second part of your superset.

Now you have finished your front-leg superset. The stopwatch will be at about 2.5–3 minutes. Take a break of between 30 seconds and 1 minute to sip some water.

Step 2: Lunges

Now get ready to work the back of the legs: the hamstring superset. This time we will do an exercise called Lunges – a superset on one leg and then the other. You'll begin with the right leg and do 8–10 weighted reps, immediately followed by 15–20 reps without weights. When that is complete, you'll move on to the left leg. This routine works the fast-twitch muscle fibres perfectly, so let's begin. Get yourself into the starting position, as shown below.

Remember, you will be holding weights in both hands straight down by the sides of your body for the first 8–10 reps. Step and bend forward with your right leg towards the ground until the right thigh is parallel to the floor. At the same time, stretch your left leg out as straight as possible behind you. Your left knee will almost touch the floor, but make sure it does not actually do so. Hold the lunge position for a second and come back up, really pushing with your right leg and squeeze those hamstrings hard. Remember to maintain your breathing: breathe in as you go down, exhale as you come up. That's one lunge done!

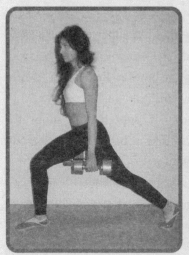 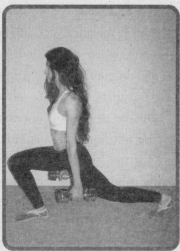

Lunges

Repeat with the same leg. Again, go down with your right thigh parallel to the floor and the left leg extended back, so your knee almost touches the ground. Hold for a second and then push back up using the right leg. That's 2 reps. Do 8–10 reps on the right side.

Once you have done the weight-bearing reps, move on to 15–20 reps without weights. Still on the right leg, complete the fast, explosive repetitions. Without a breather, move to the other leg and repeat the whole process: use weights with the first 8–10 reps, then complete the next 15–20 reps without weights.

You have now completed your back-legs hamstrings superset. A time check should show that you are 7–8 minutes into your routine. Take a 1-minute breather and sip some water.

Step 3: Dead Lift

Next up is the gluteus (bum) workout. A superset is performed with an exercise called the Dead Lift, which works the backs of the legs and dramatically lifts up the bottom. Remember to keep your breathing intact throughout this exercise.

With your heaviest dumbbells in your hands, adopt the starting position as shown. Hold the dumbbells close to your legs but not touching throughout the exercise. Starting at the top, slowly bend over until the dumbbells are at a level below your knees and your back is parallel to the floor, but no lower.

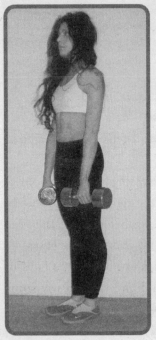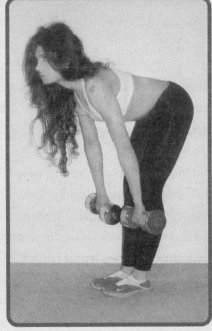

The Dead Lift

Now come back up, making sure you squeeze your bum cheeks as you rise to the standing upright position of the start. That's one rep and you will feel your bottom working. Repeat: go down slowly, keeping the weights close to your legs as shown. Hold for a second then come back up, again squeezing the cheeks as you do so.

Repeat for 8–10 reps and then switch to lighter weights and do another 15–20 reps with faster motions. This will give you a tighter, peachy behind, so really go for it!

Once you have finished the reps, you will have completed your gluteus superset and a quick time check should show between 11.5 and 12 minutes. Not bad! Now take 30 seconds to 1 minute as a breather and sip some water, then we'll do the last leg exercise.

Step 4: Calves Workout

The calves (gastrocnemius plus soleus) superset is relatively straightforward, so let's get going. Grab a set of dumbbells that are heavy enough to be testing. Hold the weights relaxed down the sides of your body, as shown overleaf.

Slowly lift both heels at the same time to balance on the front balls of your feet and toes. You will feel the calves contract as you lift. Hold for 1 second and then slowly come back down again. Repeat, slowly lifting up on to the balls of your feet and toes. Hold for 1 second and then slowly come back down again. That's 2 reps. Do 8–10 reps, keeping your breathing steady.

Now change to lighter weights and do 15–20 reps of the same

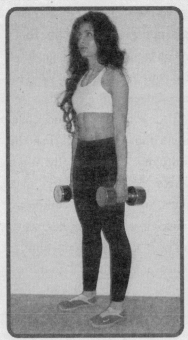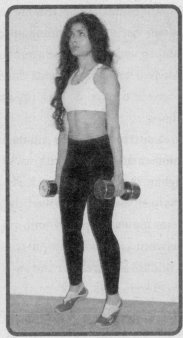

Calves Workout

movement. Once you are on your toes, come down straight away and do faster, more explosive movements, but keep them controlled. When you have finished, a time check should show 15.5–16 minutes. Take a 1-minute breather and sip some water. That's the legs done!

Step 5: Abs Superset
And now for your last superset of the day: the abdominals (or stomach) workout. Let's begin the abs superset. This time lie on the floor, place both hands behind your head, lift and bend your

knees up, with your feet flat on the floor as shown opposite. When doing your abdominal workout, remember to breathe in deeply at the start position and then breathe out as you crunch forward and your stomach muscles contract.

Prepare to do 8–10 sit-ups. Roll forward and contract your mid-section, as shown. **Don't just rock your head and neck back and forth, work the stomach. At first, you may find this movement tricky, so just work through it systematically. As you get to the crunch of each rep, hold for 1 second then lower yourself back to the starting position, all the while keeping your hands placed behind your head.**

Once you have completed your reps, drop your hands to the sides of your body, as shown. This loosens the pressure. Now raise both arms up from the floor, but still keep them by your sides. You should find this movement easier. Aim for the 15–20 reps without pause: keep crunching your abdominals until you complete the required number.

The important thing is not just to rock your head forward, but to curl or crunch round enough to cause your stomach muscles to contract. You do not have to raise yourself all the way to the knees – that is the advanced level. What you must not do, however, is to move in awkward jolts as this will do nothing for your abdominal section and can cause injury.

If you do this right, you will soon have a washboard stomach with an awesome six-pack. As the fat sheds, the beautifully worked stomach muscles will start to reveal themselves. Once you have completed your abs superset, get up and look at your stopwatch: it should read 19 minutes. Almost done!

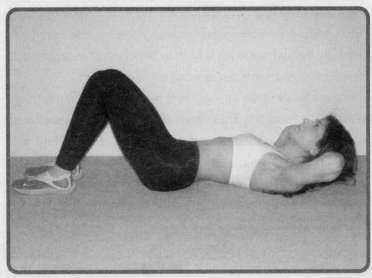

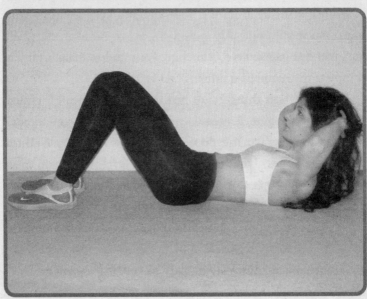

Abs Superset

Stretch to Finish

Time to stretch again to prevent Delayed Onset Muscle Soreness (DOMS). Follow the stretching plan, as before. Once you have completed it, your watch should show 20 minutes. Good job!

You have now finished the lower-body plan and, once again, released Human Growth Hormone (HGH) throughout your body through anaerobic EIGR. The amazing thing is that the extra hormones that have surged into your body are down to the workout and they will remain amplified for the next 24–48 hours, so even after your workout your body will be anti-ageing itself! You have also completed your cardiovascular session for two days in a row through the plan, which will help keep your heart strong and rejuvenate you.

Jogging Into Danger

If your current training sessions consist of aerobic workouts, running on treadmills, jogging, stair-steppers and tennis, stop right now! Aerobic exercise alone, especially high-endurance exercise like jogging, is a cause of ageing and shows a misconception of health. Of course there are benefits from jogging – it conditions the heart and makes you healthier – but it also ages you like wildfire. That's why aerobic exercise alone is not permitted on my plan.

If a personal trainer or gym instructor advises you to go jogging or to take up any other high-impact aerobic exercise for 40 minutes to an hour at a time, just say no! Note to all personal trainers and health clubs: you may want to learn from the plan and inform your clients accordingly.

Aerobic activity such as jogging, cycling or stair climbing is extremely demanding on the body. When you perform these activities, your body uses glucose for fuel at first, but when this runs out – and it does so pretty quickly – the body is forced to look elsewhere for the energy to fuel the rest of the workout and starts to consume its own healthy tissue. At this point, it targets other tissues, including muscle and skin collagen. The continuous efforts of aerobic activity and jogging alone will rapidly age your body, so you suffer degeneration in two ways: **cortisol** is released, which blocks the anti-ageing power of Human Growth Hormone, and **catabolism and muscle breakdown**, especially loss of fast-twitch fibres, occurs.

The body suffers internally when it feeds off itself and aerobic sessions usually block EIGR, instead releasing cortisol. This stress and ageing hormone causes the skin to age, wrinkles to form, the hair to thin, bones to suffer demineralisation and muscle tissue is lost so you become unhealthy and prematurely old. Now the ageing chemical cortisol is in your blood, it will block the Growth Hormone from entering.

The second reason why aerobic sport alone is so dangerous is because it breaks down your muscles as you work them and your body suffers catabolism or muscle breakdown, so fast-twitch fibres dwindle even more rapidly. You have blocked EIGR and can't flood your body with Growth Hormone. Instead, your body loses the fibres for firmness and you are left with a composition of vulnerable bones and sagging skin. That's why runners can look scrawny and skinny.

The sheer lack of anti-ageing hormones means the body

cannot protect itself from ageing and it is in an exposed state ready to be destroyed. You have fast-forwarded sarcopenia – the loss of skeletal muscle – and we already know that this is a chronic sign of ageing.

You might think that you are strengthening your heart and making yourself fitter – and, to some degree, it's true – but prolonged aerobics harms the body as it becomes loaded with cortisol and loses fast-twitch muscle fibres. Eventually, you will look older and your life expectancy could even become shortened.

The Dr Nirdosh Anti-Ageing Body Plan is the solution. It will firm, lift and provide enhanced health, while heightening feel-good endorphins and sex hormones in your body. This is your key to youth, beauty and a new, sexier you!

Chapter 6
The Dr Nirdosh Anti-Ageing Nutrition Plan

CHANGING THE WAY you eat can make you look younger, feel healthier and also live longer. Most of us eat throughout the day whenever we feel hungry and choose whatever we want. We hope to consume relatively healthy food, but eat with no real plan in mind, instead taking in what we feel suits our body type or individual requirements. However, this approach can lead to weight gain and unhappiness for millions of people because uncertainty and confusing messages about food are rife and commonly result in the wrong choices and irregular eating patterns.

If you knew that you could be part of a calculated food plan that not only guarantees that you will lose weight effortlessly, but also makes you younger and sexier, wouldn't you want to participate? The Dr Nirdosh Anti-Ageing Food Plan is a powerful, organised way to teach you what to eat.

THE MAJOR FOOD GROUPS

The food that we eat is composed of macronutrients that can be broken down into four main food groups: proteins, carbohydrates, fats, vegetables and fruit.

Proteins

Generally meats such as chicken, lamb, beef and turkey plus dairy products like milk, eggs and cheese. There are vegetarian alternatives including soya, tofu and Quorn-brand products.

When we eat, the protein is broken down into smaller peptides and amino acids. These amino acids are used as key building blocks in the formation of muscle, skin collagen, elastin, tendons, hormones, brain chemicals, hair and nails. It is necessary to include protein in your food daily – a lack of it can be dangerous. Be clear, though: not all proteins are equal and some are far better for us than others. We judge their effectiveness by the type of amino acids they contain.

The body requires 20 different such amino acids and the amazing thing is that it can generate 12 of them itself, but eight more must be supplied through diet if we are to function properly. The additional amino acids are essential for the body's survival, repair and health and are only accessible through external sources of protein, so the protein foods you eat must contain them. Foods with a higher number of amino acids in the right proportions (known as 'complete proteins') are the winners because they contain the eight essential acids that the body needs in one protein and are far superior. If you do not have sufficient amino acids, you will suffer protein deficiency. This can lead to dry, thinning hair and skin problems such as rosacea and muscle-tissue loss, as well as improper hormone synthesis.

On the Dr Nirdosh Anti-Ageing Nutrition Plan, we will focus on eating high-quality proteins that contain the eight essential amino acids in one protein food. Proteins take a long time to digest and protein metabolism requires a lot of water compared to carbohydrate and fat breakdown, so you will need to increase your water intake to 2–3 litres a day. They also keep hunger at bay as they maintain steady blood-sugar levels so you feel fuller for longer.

Carbohydrates

These are the non-meat, non-dairy foods such as breads, pasta, rice and potatoes that are associated with energy and fuel for the body, especially the brain and muscles. There are many different types of carbohydrate, including rice, cakes, sweets, chocolates, whole grains, pulses, potatoes, breads and beans. They fall into two categories:

- **Complex carbohydrates** – Starchy, natural unrefined foods that give the body a slow release of energy over sustained periods.
- **Simple carbohydrates** that give an instant energy hit like a sugar rush from refined and factory-made food.

So, complex carbohydrates are much healthier than simple ones. It's all to do with energy release and calories.

If you are hungry and have to choose between two 100-calorie carbohydrate items – a chocolate bar or a slice of wholemeal bread – which one would you pick? Most people would prefer to eat the chocolate because both contain the same number of calories, but that would be a big mistake. The chocolate bar is a simple carbohydrate, so, once it has been eaten, the body will soon experience only a short burst of energy but, when the quick energy rush runs out, the body soon becomes depleted of energy. At this point, you'll be hungry and need to eat again. Because of the up-and-down effect of energy levels, the body won't crave any old carbohydrate but will demand bad sugary ones for an instant relief. So, although you may have just eaten, your body now has a greater desire to eat bad, sugary carbohydrates, and the more you give into it, the more readily this will happen, again and again. The big mistake was choosing a food purely on the basis of calorie content with a disregard for the way the bar releases energy. Ironically, through this choice of carbohydrate, you end up feeling repeatedly hungry and will consume more calories to try to curb the pangs. You also gain weight rapidly.

If you had chosen the slice of wholemeal bread, your body would have digested it slowly and it would have made you feel satisfied for longer. The best thing is that it provides sustained energy release over a period of hours because it's a complex carbohydrate that disperses gradually. You would therefore not need to consume any more carbohydrates again for hours, so no extra calories, no extra weight gain, no deranged sugar levels, just controlled carbohydrate eating.

The wholemeal bread is better than the chocolate bar because of the rate at which carbohydrates release glucose into the blood. This is classified by the Glycaemic Index (GI), and the quicker the conversion of a carbohydrate to glucose, the higher its GI value. The lower the conversion rate, the lower the GI value and the steadier blood-sugar levels remain.

Eating too many carbohydrates, especially refined bad ones, is an easy habit to fall into and accounts for much of the obesity epidemic that we see here and in the USA.

The Danger Hormones

Eating triggers the release of hormones into the body, which receive signals that food is in the digestive system and so corresponding hormones are released to allow what you have eaten to be broken down and used. One hormone secreted in the body when food, especially carbohydrate, is consumed is insulin.

Refined carbohydrates also readily provoke the release of cortisol, which in turn affects the release of insulin. The problem is that both these danger hormones can block the vital hormone we want in our body: Growth Hormone, the anti-ageing hormone of youth.

Normally when we eat, food enters the small intestine, and the pancreas (an organ beside the stomach) releases a number of digestive hormones and enzymes, including insulin, to break down the food so it becomes absorbed in the body. Insulin is a storage hormone and a big trigger for its release is carbohydrates. It helps drive glucose into our cells to be used for energy, giving blood-glucose levels the chance to stabilise.

Overeating carbohydrates, especially the wrong sort, has bred a civilisation suffering from insulin resistance – a dangerous borderline diabetic condition. The body responds to the frequent carbohydrate indulgences by producing more and more insulin (hyperinsulinaemia) because cells in the body have become unresponsive to the insulin present. There is nothing to clear the sugar from the blood or to drive it into our cells, especially into the muscles and the brain, and, when these do not have enough energy, they become lethargic. Excess glucose floats around the blood and causes havoc to our organs. Left for long enough, it can gnaw away and rot them, causing damage to the skin, eyes and nerves.

The deranged blood-sugar levels also cause recurrent food cravings, a cycle of eating without feeling satisfied and mood swings. Surplus insulin leads to rapid weight gain as it increases free fatty acids in the blood and fat deposition, especially around the stomach. This can lead to clinical obesity.

When insulin resistance is accompanied by lethargy, hunger pangs, mood swings, weight gain, raised blood pressure and irritability, this often means that the body has developed a serious medical disorder called metabolic syndrome. If you relate to these feelings, then you may be suffering from insulin resistance and unknowingly have full-blown metabolic syndrome. This can easily progress to Type 2 diabetes and increased risk of coronary heart disease, both of which are killers. That's why you should avoid junk and processed foods: usually fat-laden and sugary, they release simple carbohydrates fast.

Refined carbohydrates, which include white bread, ready meals, pasta, white rice and noodles, can cause further medical complications including the release of cortisol, the bad ageing hormone we talked about earlier. This can cause acne, skin inflammation and poor health of the inner organs. In contrast, most centenarians – irrespective of which part of the world they come from – usually have low insulin and stable blood-sugar levels.

The Dr Nirdosh Anti-Ageing Nutrition Plan permits only unrefined complex carbohydrates: wholegrain and wholemeal carbohydrates such as brown rice, couscous, beans and pulses. These keep blood-sugar levels steady and help avoid insulin resistance, as well as excess cortisol release. The selected foods are rich in vitamins, especially B vitamins, minerals and other nutritiously beneficial components. They take time to digest, so the body feels fuller for longer as your desire to eat more is quashed and you feel satisfied.

Vegetables and Fruit

Sometimes vegetables and fruit are considered carbohydrates, although their main job is to provide the body with essential vitamins, minerals and antioxidants rather than to be a source of energy. Since most are low in sugar, they won't cause imbalances. Instead, these nutritious foods provide highly potent protecting and repairing nutrients that the body needs to stay young.

The fruit and vegetables permitted on the Dr Nirdosh Anti-Ageing Nutrition Plan are fibrous and not high in sugars. They also top the league when it comes to fighting free radicals and neutralise the cell-damaging toxins that age the body. Some of the fruit and vegetables on the plan are also negative-calorie foods, which means they require more calories to break down than they actually contain so you lose calories while you eat!

Negative-calorie fruit and vegetables include celery, lettuce, cucumber, onion, garlic, radishes, cress, cranberries, raspberries and grapefruit.

Fats

We assume fats are bad for you because we associate the word with becoming fat, but it's not always true. The body needs certain essential fats and these must be supplied through what we eat.

There are two types of fat: saturated and unsaturated. Let's take a look at them both:

- **Saturated fats** are usually solid fats, which are dangerous and to be avoided. Once consumed, they stick to vital organs such as the heart and clog arteries so you risk cardiovascular disease. They are commonly found in fatty meats and full-fat dairy produce, including butter, margarine, lard, cream, full-fat milk and full-fat cheese. Saturated fats also include trans fats and hydrogenated fats, both of which are hazardous to health.
- **Unsaturated fats** are usually liquid at room temperature and include several oils. As well as being found in olive oil, they are contained in many nuts, avocados and oily fish. They contain essential fats, which cannot be created by the body and must be supplied through diet.

Essential fats form part of the lipid wall, the surrounding of every cell in our body. They are also required in hormone metabolism, and fat itself cushions our organs, including our skin, to protect our bones and muscles from injury. Essential fats form part of the myelin sheath – the protective coating that surrounds the nerves in the brain, too.

Fats are also required in the body to allow absorption and transport of vital fat-soluble nutrients including vitamins A, D, E and K. However, excess fats are dangerous, especially those that accumulate around the mid-abdominal region and the visceral fat surrounding our organs. Excess fat predisposes to cardiovascular disease and increases the risk of certain cancers.

My plan focuses on unsaturated essential fats such as omega 3 and 6, as well as the vital but non-essential omega 9. This might sound like a bit of a contradiction but omega 9 is referred to as non-essential because the body can manufacture it providing that the raw materials are present in adequate quantities. However, making omega 9 available via nutritional or supplementary sources ensures that this important fatty acid is always there to work in line with the others to boost skin appearance, smooth lines and keep the complexion in a well-moisturised state.

These fats help to signal fullness for long periods and won't cause an imbalance in blood-sugar or insulin levels. The acids also encourage the body to burn fat better, helping you to stay lean.

EATING CAUSES AGEING

Perhaps you eat whenever you feel hungry or maybe you find it difficult to stop. You could be eating good-quality nutrients or foods laden in fat and sugar. Either way, your eating habits now are almost certainly incorrect and are speeding up your ageing process.

The reason we age when we eat is not just due to the foods we consume but also to the frequency of our meals. Humans eat too many times a day and take in far too many calories, which fast-forwards ageing in the face and body. Every time we eat like this, we turn the digestive system into a machine for ageing. Food may fuel us and give us satisfaction, but it also elevates ageing through bad-hormone release and premature apoptosis (early cell death).

Whenever we eat, the body has to break the food down into useable calories. The more frequent the meals we consume, the more times the body's digestive process must kick in to digest the food. When we eat again and again, this process also occurs again and again. The relentlessly overworked digestive system turns the body into a metabolic churning machine, which eventually results in overworked cells. The cells tire until finally they become exhausted and die. This leads to premature ageing.

You may be thinking: that's not me because I eat high-quality calories and I'm slim. But have you ever wondered why your face and body are beginning to age fast and you're looking haggard? It's because slim people also can have bad dietary habits. Just because you eat the right amount of calories, your body isn't necessarily healthy. The calories may be correct, but your eating method may not be. Eating every two to three hours can cause frequent releases of insulin and the stress hormone cortisol, as well as overworking your cells and exposing you to ageing toxins.

MAKING THE CHANGE

The clever thing about the Dr Nirdosh Anti-Ageing Nutrition Plan is that, from now on, the way you eat will make you look younger and live longer by harnessing the power of Growth Hormone-enhancing foods and activating the anti-ageing gene SIRT 1. The first principle of the plan is to eat Growth Hormone-enhancing foods to place the body in a state that supports cellular repair. This hormone decreases fat, enhances muscle tissue, increases bone density, boosts immunity and preserves brain function. Other benefits include an increase in skin collagen, sexual libido and facial youth; it also lowers bad cholesterol, raises strength and the ability to exercise, as well as improving sleep. This is the master of all hormones and we will increase it with the Dr Nirdosh Anti-Ageing Nutrition Plan, as well as through specialised fasting.

At mealtimes, the foods eaten will help stimulate the release of anti-ageing hormones and we will achieve this through the right nutrition that acts as Growth Hormone Secretagogues (GHSs) – in other words, foods that enhance leanness and youth by signalling the release of this hormone into the body.

Substances such as certain amino acids act on the hypothalamic-pituitary system in the brain, provoking it to release Growth Hormone into the blood. This is carried to our organs to help keep our skin and body blooming with youth. The trick is to find the foods that are the highest stimulants of Growth Hormone release. The best GHSs are those that contain all eight essential amino acids, as these have the most power to stimulate its release. The amino acids arginine and ornithine are particularly powerful GHSs. Others include glutamine, lysine and glycine. Foods rich in these natural enhancers of Growth Hormone include:

- Fish
- Eggs
- Lean meats
- Poultry
- Low-fat dairy products

Eating these on the food plan helps stimulate the production of anti-ageing hormones, which encourages lost skin collagen fibres to be rebuilt to help firm the face again and fight wrinkles while tightening and dropping fat from the body.

Complete amino protein food sources contain all eight essential amino acids, including those that stimulate Human Growth Hormone release, thereby helping to make the skin and body look younger. This enhances the body's immunity and sexual function so that it starts to become naturally youthful from within. We will be eating these foods at every meal.

THE ANTI-AGEING GENE

You have a gene in your body that's capable of making you live longer yet most people rarely use it. The Dr Nirdosh Anti-Ageing Nutrition Plan reactivates this wonder gene through food. Animals regularly use this method to eat and it can increase their lifespan by up to 30 per cent. If we humans activated this gene, we could live for two extra decades.

Most humans don't know about the gene – or, like my celebrity clients, they do know and prefer to keep the secret to themselves. The problem is that, with today's sedentary lifestyles and overeating, the anti-ageing gene has become dormant over the years and is probably seldom activated, if at all. My plan will awaken this gene through a unique way of eating that helps block ageing. You'll eat to live longer!

The food plan is developed to turn on the anti-ageing gene SIRT 1 and enable the body to put a major brake on cell functions and ageing. It will achieve this amazing feat through the powers of fasting and calorie restriction, which will give your body the automatic bionic power to halt fast-paced ageing, quickly shift excess weight and enable you to live longer.

Fasting also releases Growth Hormone and blocks the ageing hormone. I first encountered its unique powers when I was a child performer and was rushed from one location to another without any food. In the process, I realised three things: I never ran out of energy, I didn't need to eat again for hours and I remained sharp and alert throughout my fasts.

I decided that, while I was performing, I would follow this fasting plan. It made my body feel great and it adjusted quickly to the new regime. This was different from starvation because I ate nutritious food at regular intervals. I left gaps of up to six hours before I would eat again but I didn't understand why it felt so good for me at the time. In fact, I could go for hours without suffering hunger pangs or energy deficiencies. It was later while working as a doctor that I decided to research further and discovered the medical components of what had occurred during these short periods of fasting and controlled food intake. That is when I found out about SIRT 1, the anti-ageing gene.

So we know that eating excess calories elevates ageing as the body goes into overdrive and starts the premature activity of cell damage that leads to their untimely death. However, we can also reverse or slow down this reaction through fasting and not overeating. Preserving the lifespan of every cell is vital – we can conserve and even prolong this through fasting and calorie control so that cells work less often and can even live longer, thus slowing down ageing in the process.

SIX – THE MAGIC NUMBER

On the Dr Nirdosh Anti-Ageing Nutrition Plan, you will fast with six-hour gaps between each calorie-controlled meal. You might think that fasting means no eating, but the good news is that you will be eating three satisfying, nutritious meals every day. However, this plan will give you anti-ageing benefits that not everyone gets – you'll be eating the way that many A-list celebrities have been doing for decades. My celebrity clients know how food can help you get great results, and now you too can discover their secret. **Before you start my plan, please check with your doctor that there are no contraindications to fasting for six-hour periods.**

The best thing about the plan is that you don't need to change much of what you may be accustomed to eating, while eating foods that are tasty and anti-ageing. You also get to drink wine! Luxuries and pleasures you may be familiar with will still be part of your life and the plan will not turn it upside down.

There is a magical effect to fasting: the body recognises a fasting period and calorie restriction, and fasting tricks it into mild fear and puts it in a defensive state so it biologically stresses to save cells and tissues from damage. During this period, the body turns on the superpower anti-ageing gene, SIRT 1.

In Western civilisation, the body never has to endure really dangerous fears such as a water shortage, excessive cold, food deficiency and the like. Because of this, it never has its safeguard on, making it vulnerable to damage and premature ageing. However, if the body thinks there is a dangerous food-deficient period ahead, it will quickly put up a strong defence barrier against ageing.

Animals use fasting as a safety mechanism: when they are ill, they stop eating as they know instinctively that this allows the immune system to kick back strongly and deliver healing. But humans rarely fast and, when we are unwell, we sometimes even eat more and this can actually increase illness. Eating causes the release of stress hormones including cortisol and insulin, so the more frequently you indulge, the more you age. While these stress hormones are being secreted, the anti-ageing ones are being suppressed.

Through fasting and calorie restriction, you can activate the secret anti-ageing gene inside your body, instructing it to stop the age clock. It does this through autolysis – where the body draws on its own fat reserves for fuel and also uses nutrients in storage such as the fat-soluble vitamins A, E, D and K. At the same time, it also rids itself of cells that have suffered previous damage, clearing them away to leave behind a cleaner, healthier body with cells in a good, undamaged condition. This system helps to slow down early apoptosis (slow cell death). Since the body thinks that it will need all its resources after the fasting and reduced-calorie period, it goes into overdrive to protect its cells. Dr Nirdosh's Anti-Ageing Nutrition Plan also helps decrease oxidation and free-radical production, all accelerators of ageing.

When you fast, you will notice some symptoms such as a runny nose as mucous production increases. The body will also excrete toxins, so your urine may appear darker as the kidneys eliminate them. Metabolically and hormonally, the body alters: insulin levels decrease and blood-sugar levels are lowered, enhancing Human Growth Hormone release. This fasting and calorie-control principle provides a double de-ageing effect by helping the body turn on SIRT 1 and secrete Human Growth Hormone.

Fasting increases the breakdown of fat, especially fat surrounding our organs, as this is far more dangerous than fat between our skin and muscle. Fat here creates pro-inflammatory chemicals called cytokines and prostaglandins that have pre-cancerous abilities. Through fasting, the body will become efficient at using fat for fuel, which leads to rapid weight loss, and the conservation of collagen and elastin will help to improve facial lift and firmness. Immune strength is also raised and the digestive system has a chance to stay young as the body eliminates hazardous waste from the liver and kidneys.

Be clear, however, that this is not starvation but fasting: voluntary abstinence from food. We will deliberately leave six-hour pauses between meals to activate the anti-ageing gene SIRT 1 and enhance secretion of Human Growth Hormone. At mealtimes, we will feed the body with essential amino acids and micronutrients – potent doses of vitamins, minerals and antioxidants will provide vital raw materials to help repair age damage and enhance the body's resistance to further ageing. This unique nutrition plan ensures that, both during meals and between them, the body is prepared to enter a maximum anti-ageing zone.

LOSE WEIGHT FAST

Your changed eating habits mean that you will now lose weight quickly, dropping up to three dress sizes in just six weeks. You'll have a new, sexier body primed to stay defined and youthful for years to come. So, get ready to begin the top-secret food programme that I have developed over many years and prescribe daily to numerous high-profile clients. My wonder nutritional plan stops wrinkles, slows down ageing, reshapes the body to look stunningly sexy and produces a much more youthful face.

You may have tried diets and fads before, but this is a true lifestyle change and a new way of eating targeted solely on making your body counteract ageing from the inside out. Through the plan, you will learn how to slow down apoptosis, so your cells live longer and discover how your body will release Human Growth Hormone – the hormone that gives you back your youthful looks and fixes a time-damaged face.

Remember, you must leave six-hour fasts between meals, so, if you eat breakfast at 7am, then your next meal will be at 1pm and the final one at 7pm. If you have breakfast at 8am, follow it with your next meal at 2pm and the last at 8pm. The latest you must have breakfast is 9am. That way you will not be consuming your last meal too late at night. If you lapse during the eating plan, don't worry too much – just don't use it as an excuse to go off the rails or to stop the plan. It's OK to have a blip – just don't make it a regular occurrence.

Start Timeframes

	(A)	(B)	(C)
Breakfast (meal one)	7am	8am	9am
Midday (meal two)	1pm	2pm	3pm
Evening (meal three)	7pm	8pm	9pm

You can follow any of the three timeframes (A, B or C) on any one day, but you must allow a six-hour break in between, as the fasting and calorie-restriction work to activate the anti-ageing gene and enhance anti-ageing Growth Hormone secretion.

PORTION SIZES

Uncertainty over portion sizes can lead to overeating and excess calories, but on the food plan that follows you will get a general overview by working in cup sizes (use a cup that holds approx 250ml/8fl oz of fluid). For example, if you choose chicken as your protein portion, then you will need approximately 1 cup of chopped chicken – about the size of an average chicken breast or one thigh. If you miss a meal or stray from the plan, do not worry: just make sure from your next meal that you jump back on to the plan.

At first, your body may find the new regime slightly confusing, but it will quickly fall into place and soon you'll only need to eat at the given times. As your body adjusts, you'll notice that the calorie reduction is working perfectly. You will not suffer hunger pangs because you will still be eating three meals a day. Any cravings will be kept at bay with slow energy-release carbohydrates that will help you get to your next meal easily.

WATER

Drink plenty of water, at least 2–3 litres (3½–5¼ pints) each day. It's one of the most important nutrients since the human body contains 45–70 per cent water. As your muscle tissue increases, so too does the need for water. Muscle tissue and skin contain about 70 per cent water, while blood has up to 85 per cent.

It's easy to confuse thirst with hunger so you can end up eating food instead of replenishing fluids. On the plan, you'll be drinking water with every meal and in between.

FOOD GROUPS

On the plan, you'll select an item from each food group below (A, B, C and D). Follow the guidelines in Group E for anti-ageing drinks. You are also permitted a choice of anti-ageing condiments with every meal.

- **Group A: Proteins** Growth Hormone-boosting foods
- **Group B: Carbohydrates** Slow energy-release foods
- **Group C: Vegetables and Fruit** Nutrient-rich antioxidants, vitamins and minerals
- **Group D: Fats** Essential Fatty Acids (EFAs) – vital body functioning fats
- **Group E: Anti-Ageing Drinks**
- **Additional: Anti-Ageing Condiments**

Groups A, B, C and D are vital. Group A feeds the body with Growth Hormone-enhancing foods that provide the complete amino acids to reinject youth. Group B gives the right amount of energy for the body to survive the six-hour fasts. Group C provides vital nutrients, antioxidants, vitamins and minerals so the body maintains optimum health, vitality and repairs itself, while Group D gives the tiny amounts of essential fat necessary to help protect your organs.

Group E is a little treat, giving you a choice of a few healthy drinks with every meal. They taste great and help speed up the results of the plan.

Remember, you will be eating to anti-age and transform your body. My food plan will help you lose a dramatic amount of weight and make your body younger internally, so that, externally, you will reap the results.

(Note: we will use a cup that can hold 250ml (8fl oz) of liquid or flaked/chopped ingredients.)

Group A: Anti-Ageing Proteins

(1 cup with each meal)

• Tuna • Halibut • Bass • Herring • Salmon • Mackerel • Sardines • Liver/kidneys • Lean lamb • Veal • Lean beef • Turkey • Chicken • Goose/wild duck/pheasant • Venison • Guinea fowl • 4 egg whites/1 yolk • Low-fat milk (skimmed)• Low-fat fromage frais • Quail eggs • Low-fat goats' milk • Low-fat cottage cheese • Low-fat Cheddar • Low-fat Parmesan • Low-fat Gruyère • Low-fat mozzarella • Low-fat feta • Low-fat ricotta • Low-fat Edam • Monkfish • Low-fat halloumi • Vegetarian meats • Soya protein • Tofu • Low-fat, low-salt ham • Low-fat, low-salt bacon or lean pork • Quorn • Prawns • Oysters • Fish eggs (roe)/ caviar • Snails • Clams • Crab meat • Scallops • Squid

Group B: Vegetables and Fruit

(½ cup of veg and ½ cup of fruit with each meal – raw is best!)
• Vine/beef /cherry tomatoes • Lambs'/Romaine (Cos) lettuce •
Kale • Bok choi • Lima beans • Alfalfa sprouts • Rocket • Brussels
sprouts • Beetroot • Spinach • Leeks • Onions • Radishes • Red
cabbage • Broccoli • Artichoke hearts • Peppers • Broad beans •
Petits pois • Raw carrots • Seaweed • Collard greens • Green beans
• Cucumber

• Watermelon/Cantaloupe • Cherries • Black/red seeded grapes •
Strawberries • Pomegranate • Blueberries • Raspberries •
Blackberries • Black plums • Sour green apples • Passionfruit •
Goji/acai berries • Cranberries • Kiwis • Mandarins • Grapefruit

Group C: Anti-Ageing Carbohydrates

(½ cup size with your first two meals of the day, but no Group C
for your last meal)
•Wheatgerm • Brown rice • Couscous • Barley • Bran • Oatmeal •
Russet potatoes • Yams • Red adzuki beans • Kidney beans • Pinto
beans • Black-eyed peas • Wild black rice • Lentils • Butternut
squash • Unripe banana • Wholemeal bread (maximum of 2 slices
daily) • Celeriac • Pumpkin • Red rice • Wholemeal pita

Group D: Anti-Ageing Fats

(1 teaspoon with each meal for oils, or a palm-size portion of
nuts, seeds, etc.)
• Olive oil • Palm oil • Coconut oil • Rice bran oil • Corn oil •
Rapeseed oil • 4–5 olives • Almonds • Flax seeds • Brazil nuts •

Walnuts • Pumpkin seeds • Pure peanut butter • Avocado • Cashews • Sesame seeds (1 teaspoon) • Macadamia nuts • Pine nuts • Pecans

Group E: Anti-Ageing Drinks

(approximately a 200ml serving for each)
• Water (2–3 litres/3½–5¼ pints a day) • Green tea (plus lemon slice) 2 to 3 cups per day) • Red wine (3 glasses each week) • Tomato juice • Herbal tea (no sugar) • Red/black tea (2 cups per day max, 1 with breakfast) • Rooibos tea • Dandelion coffee • PM fat-reduced cocoa/no sugar • Freshly squeezed vegetable juice • Freshly squeezed mandarin juice (2 mandarins) • Freshly squeezed grapefruit juice (1 grapefruit) • Sparkling mineral water, still mineral water, filtered water or tap water with freshly squeezed lemon or lime juice

Additional: Anti-Ageing Condiments

(Choose any of the following to accompany and flavour meals. You can have an unlimited amount of condiments, either dried or fresh – just ensure that they are not preserved in oil or sugar)
• Cinnamon • Pepper • Lemon juice • Lime juice • Cayenne (chilli pepper) • Vinegar (malt, wine or balsamic are particularly good)• Rosemary • Garlic • Ginger • Thyme • Basil • Parsley • Cumin • Oregano • Mint • Dill • Watercress

You are not permitted food from Group C (anti-ageing carbohydrates) for your last meal of the day. Eating these slow-release foods just before bedtime means you won't work off the calories after your meal, so promoting weight gain.

Certain things are banned on the food plan:

- Cigarettes
- Chocolate
- Sweets
- White breads and rice
- Pasta
- Fizzy drinks or sugary soft drinks
- Coffee
- Processed foods
- Crisps and similar snacks
- Fast food/takeaways
- Ready meals
- Alcohol other than red wine
- Butter and margarine

You can use a diary to write down your meal plans so you can see in advance what you will be eating each day. Keep the information with you so you know when and what you are eating.

THE FIVE-MEAL MYTH

A lot of people graze through the day, eating every two to three hours. Most of them end up eating five meals each day, commonly choosing three full-size ones and two to three snacks. There's a mistaken belief that eating five smaller meals a day is good for you. It has been stated that nibbling slowly throughout the day and spacing your calorie intake over five meals is a healthy way to eat to stabilise your metabolism; however, this actually overburdens the body and causes it to overwork. Because it is continuously receiving food, it is constantly working hard to digest and absorb it, a process that creates harmful free radicals as a by-product, so accelerating ageing. Also, constant eating causes insulin levels to frequently surge, suppressing vital Growth Hormone release.

YOUTH IN A GLASS OF WINE

The plan permits you to drink three units of red wine a week. Good scientific evidence suggests that red wine contains resveratrol, which can help trigger SIRT 1 (the longevity gene) to work, while also acting as a potent antioxidant to neutralise ageing toxins. Resveratrol is a powerful molecule found in foods such as red grapes and berries, which are ingredients in red wine. So, red wine should be your treat drink of choice on evenings out, but, remember, wine is also loaded with sugars and calories, so stick to three glasses a week, no more – and not in one go!

EXAMPLE MEAL PLANS
Breakfast Options

- 4 lean turkey rashers or low-salt, low-fat bacon, 1 grilled tomato, ½ cup black seeded grapes, 1 wholemeal toast or a small unripe banana.
- Omelette (made with 4 egg whites, 1 yolk), ½ courgette, ½ tomato, sprinkling grated low-fat Cheddar, 1 wholemeal pita and ½ cup raspberries.
- ½ cup unrefined porridge oats, 250ml (8fl oz) skimmed milk,

3 egg whites (or 1 scoop whey protein powder), 1 teaspoon peanut butter, ½ cup raw grated carrots and ½ cup blueberries.

- 250ml (8fl oz) low-fat fromage frais, sprinkling walnuts, ½ cantaloupe and ½ cup raw grated carrots.

- 2 lean sausages (preferably turkey or chicken), 2 eggs scrambled (1 yolk, 2 whites), ½ can plum tomato mixed with ½ can pinto beans and ½ cup pomegranate seeds.

- Poached egg with salmon on slices of grilled russet potatoes, mozzarella, cherry tomatoes, beetroot, cucumber, dill and 1 sour green apple, sliced.

- Great anti-ageing breakfast drinks: green tea, freshly squeezed grapefruit and mandarin juice or tomato juice.

Lunch Ideas

- Chicken, beef or ham sandwich made with 1 slice wholemeal fresh bread (sliced diagonally), filled with a salad of beef tomatoes, avocado, spinach leaves, lemon juice and 1 teaspoon low-fat fromage frais as dressing.

- ½ cup Mediterranean-style couscous, with red and green diced peppers, juice of ½ fresh orange and ½ fresh lime, 1 kiwi (diced), 1 x 185g (6¼oz) can tuna in brine (drained) and 1 teaspoon olive oil.

- Mackerel and wild black or red rice salad (½ cup cooked rice), ½ cup red cabbage (shredded) and 1 diced black plum, basil and peppercorns.

- 1 homemade lamb or venison burger in wholemeal pita, with a salad of tomatoes, radish, alfalfa sprouts with passion fruit and chopped chilli as dressing.

- Egg salad (2 egg whites, 1 yolk), mixed with low-fat ricotta, ½ cup roasted diced potatoes, ½ cup blackberries and ½ cup rocket, plus seasoning to taste.
- Prawns mixed with ½ cup adzuki or kidney beans, pine nuts, watercress, sliced vine tomatoes, 4–5 pitted olives and black grapes. (For a vegetarian option, swap the prawns for low-fat cottage cheese.)

Dinner Choices

- Beef steak, ½ cup lima beans, onion gravy, diced radishes and a medley of mixed berries with 1 teaspoon low-fat fromage frais or yoghurt for dessert, topped with pecan nuts.
- ½ baby roast chicken or guinea fowl garnished with garlic, basil and seasoning, with fresh tomato and blueberry salsa.
- Halibut shallow-fried in 1 teaspoon rice bran oil with garlic, salt, lemon juice, vinegar, pepper and almond flakes, plus 2 diced olives and accompanied by steamed green beans or petits pois and watermelon for dessert.
- Bouillabaisse of shellfish, monkfish with chopped leeks and salmon, followed by a mix of low-fat ricotta, strawberries, mandarin and pumpkin seeds for dessert.
- Slow-roasted lean cut of lamb seasoned with rock salt, peppercorns and rosemary, served with kale or brussel sprouts, liver gravy, fresh mint sauce and tiramisu minus biscotti and alcohol (made with low-fat ricotta, decaffeinated coffee and almond flakes, lightly dusted with sifted pure cocoa powder).
- Grilled or pan-fried veal or game (first seasoned with

oregano, rock salt and pepper), with steamed artichoke hearts and ½ cup cherries for dessert.

Special Meal Tips

- For an anti-ageing mashed-potato equivalent, use butternut squash, pumpkin, yam or celeriac.
- Having a hectic day at work and no time to pre-prepare lunch? Don't worry: pick a low-fat sandwich like ham, prawn, fresh salmon, egg salad or chicken salad from any food hall. Take the two halves of the sandwich and discard one side of the bread from each. Now combine the two halves containing the filling so you eat half the bread and double the filling. Low-fat, sugar-free yoghurt and an apple makes an easy dessert.
- Be careful with readymade dressings – they contain a lots of hidden calories.
- Is your sweet tooth kicking in? Take a couple of squares of chocolate that's at least 80 per cent cocoa solids, but don't make this a daily habit! It will also provide you with some anti-ageing polyphenols (antioxidants).
- Maybe you're getting cravings? Carry some plain nuts around with you to stabilise your blood-sugar levels and dissolve hunger pangs. Only a small handful, though! They're high in nutrients, including protein and Essential Fatty Acids.
- When you're on the move, between meetings or maybe your lunchtime is delayed due to a deadline and you're feeling hungry, avoid crisps and chocolates and stock up on beef jerky instead. This saviour snack is high in protein and low in

fat, so it's ideal on the anti-ageing programme. Beef jerky is my handbag buddy!

- Add black pepper to your meals – it's high in chromium which helps stabilise blood-sugar levels.

- Got back from work late and famished? To avoid reaching for the toast, keep some ready-boiled eggs, vegetable crudités, chicken or meat slices such as low-salt ham in your fridge to suppress your appetite while you cook your anti-ageing evening meal.

- Maybe you're out in a restaurant but you don't know what to choose to stay on track. Ensure you skip Group C carbohydrates and go for fish, meats or vegetarian alternatives with fresh veggies. For dessert, pick a fruit or yoghurt option. Mousses and sorbets generally have less fat and calories than most cakes. And, yes, you can have that glass of red wine!

- Instead of sugar, use sucralose as sweetener, but don't make this a frequent habit! It is an artificially manufactured product that creates a sweet-tooth habit.

- Low-fat fromage frais or low-fat ricotta are great as mayonnaise or dressing equivalents and very versatile, too, as they can be used for savoury or dessert options. Plus, they're high in protein.

- No time to cook? Stir-fries are a quick and easy anti-ageing treat. Choose chicken, turkey or fish and mix with your choice of vegetables, like broccoli, peppers and seaweed. Add some bean sprouts, cashews and a dash of soy sauce. Dinner in 10 minutes!

- When you think you're starving and you're about to grab the closest food to hand, stop and drink a glass of water. The most common mistake is to confuse thirst with hunger and this tiny switch will help you lose loads of weight.

- Watch out for hidden sugar and fats in products like ham, e.g. honey roast varieties.

- Choose decaffeinated coffee over caffeinated ones which raise cortisol and insulin levels.

- A great high-antioxidant tea alternative is rooibos tea and a totally natural caffeine-free coffee alternative is dandelion coffee.

- Green tea is an excellent anti-ager as it gives you beauty, youth and a slim body. The favourite drink of supermodels, it contains powerful antioxidants – Epigallocatechin Gallates (EGCGs) and speeds up fat loss. It also contains theanine – an amino acid that helps to suppress the release of cortisol and acts on the brain to change brainwave activity to a calmer, but alert state. Drink two to three cups a day.

- Stay clear of smoothies and fruit juices (other than the ones made with ingredients listed in the anti-ageing condiments and drinks plan) because both are high in sugars.

- Avoid butters and margarine as they often contain trans or hydrogenated fats, which are bad for you as they can lead to clogging of the arteries, raise cholesterol and increase the risk of heart disease and stroke.

- Sparkling mineral water with a dash of fresh lemon or mandarin juice makes a great accompaniment to an evening meal. It also makes an ideal substitute for fizzy drinks.

Chapter 7

The Dr Nirdosh Anti-Ageing Skincare Plan

MILLIONS OF PEOPLE use an array of different skincare products on their faces. Some simply slap on a basic moisturiser, while others seek a wonder cream in the hope of looking decades younger. What a lot of people don't know, however, is that, when creams are used correctly as treatments for specific skin types and age profiles, wonderful results can be achieved.

The biggest mistake is to discard a cream when it proves not to show any real change. You must consider skincare as a treatment to stick with, not just a run-of-the-mill ritual. Just as you would treat a wound with care, skincare for ageing should be given the same respect. You are treating the face to heal and correct damage in the form of fine lines, wrinkles and sagging skin, and your sole intention is to make repairs. Do you think just a small amount of a basic cream used infrequently will produce the required results? Of course not!

Healing any kind of wound or scar takes time and a concerted effort, which may include a change of diet, a progressive supplement prescription plan and changes of dressings. Skincare works similarly, so you need a meticulous treatment master plan that will work to heal and protect age-damaged skin. But how do you formulate a plan for your skin type? The Dr Nirdosh Anti-Ageing Skincare Plan is tailored to be a clever, individual blueprint to beat ageing.

The face is one of the first parts of the body to show telltale signs of ageing and it's here that we try our best to conceal the evidence. To minimise and slow down facial ageing, we must pay a great deal of attention to the face and invest in a good skincare regime. If we supply the right type of treatments and give facial skin the time and attention it deserves, it will react by fixing – and even reversing – the signs of ageing.

Ageing is not pre-determined, as most people seem to think. You can slow it down to ensure that you age gracefully. Naturally, you hope that it's not going to happen prematurely, resulting in you looking older than your years. This depressing attitude might have held true some 40 years ago, but it no longer stands. We have advanced dramatically since then and skin science proves that we can hold ageing at bay, no matter what our real age, provided we take the right measures. These will allow the skin to regain lost youth, just like any other part of the body.

Ageing is more noticeable in problematic areas such as around the eyes, where crow's feet, dark circles and bags can appear. Then there are jowls, thinning lips and turkey neck. You may suffer from some of these and wonder how to address them.

The Dr Nirdosh Anti-Ageing Skincare Plan will give you a specific regime for your age and skin type, while addressing each concern so you know that you are feeding your skin with the best molecules and correct nutrients to fight back. The results will be stunning. For the first time you can be confident that, finally, you have the right skincare routine. You'll know the products you need, which gives you total control of a proper treatment plan.

You must protect your skin daily and it's never too late to start. When you combine this plan with the Dr Nirdosh exercise and nutrition schemes, you will reap the benefits of hormonal changes to your body, making you look younger and more uplifted. We must capitalise on this by providing the facial cells with essential products such as anti-ageing creams, cleansers, toners, eye-fixing creams, specialist serums and washes. Facial skin has to combat elements such as weather and pollution and we must protect it from the many factors that accelerate ageing, too. So why does the face age?

SMOKING

Smoking is a major culprit. It disfigures beautiful skin and accelerates ageing dramatically. When 20-year-old skin is monitored under a microscope, you can see the onset of deep wrinkles and lines. Imagine what it must be like if you smoke 10 or more cigarettes a day for the next decade. Eventually, the face will appear creased and saggy; it will also take on a leathery look with a yellowish tinge from the harsh chemicals.

All this happens because each cigarette contains thousands of harmful toxins that enter the bloodstream and work their way around the internal organs. Every puff destroys skin's infrastructure, oxygen levels are reduced, blood vessels become constricted and the skin is starved of nutrients, especially vitamin C. This hampers the production of collagen and elasticity.

I always tell my celebrity clients that, if they are to succeed on my plan, they must stop smoking immediately and completely. There's a glimmer of hope that, as soon as anyone does stop, their complexion quickly improves and they start to see a fading of lines as the face begins to heal and detoxify from all those fumes. The problem is that celebrities are often spotted flaunting a cigarette and this has been the case from the movie stars of yesteryear to today's A-list. But there's nothing cool about smoking – just look at the government warnings that it kills.

DEATH IN THE SUN

Without the sun we could not survive and would suffer numerous illnesses such as rickets, a bone disease related to vitamin D deficiency. Yet the sun is also one of the most common causes of ageing.

A tanned skin is deemed beautiful, but it's also a death trap. Skin cancer is one of the most common cancers today and the primary cause is the sun and excessive tanning. Sun ageing occurs as a result of damage by ultraviolet rays. It usually happens over a period of many, many years as the UV rays affect natural collagen reproduction in the skin and break down existing fibres and elasticity. This is ageing in overdrive: we need collagen and elastin to plump up the skin and make it stand firm.

Long bouts of sun damage cause sagging, deep wrinkles and serious loss of elasticity. Excessive sun worshipping also creates hyperpigmentation patches – seen as freckles or sunspots, as well as dry, coarse and loose skin. The good news is that the skin does have a protective mechanism to absorb some UV rays in the form of melanin, the pigment that gives our outer layer its colour. However, the lighter the skin tone, the less melanin it carries, so fair Caucasian skin is most vulnerable to damage.

Normally, melanin absorbs UV radiation and, as it does so, the skin becomes darker, producing a gradual tan. When you suffer sunburn, the rays have overloaded the skin so much that you have first-degree burns, with blistering and aching. Long-term exposure is closely linked to the various forms of skin cancer: malignant melanoma, basal and squamous cell carcinomas (SCC). All aspects of tanning, whether gradual or as severe as sunburn, are seriously dangerous and make us age, so tanning is not permitted on the skincare plan.

AGEING IN THE AIR

Harsh environmental factors such as pollution also trigger ageing in the face without us even noticing and leave pimples, blackheads, lines and dull-looking skin in their wake. The rays in pollution can penetrate deeper into the skin than those from the sun, causing far-reaching internal disruption.

The skin ages a little every day and it's ironic that the air we breathe to keep us alive is the same air that can eventually lead to our death. It works like this: take an apple and cut it in half; place one half in a sealed container and leave the other on a table in a room at normal temperature for two hours. When you come back to the fruit, the half in the container will show little, if any, damage, while the one left in the open air will have already browned as it slowly rots away. It has suffered oxidative damage.

Over many years, our skin suffers in the same way. We progressively look older as polluted and unbalanced oxygen damages its surface, just like the brown half of the apple. This is why Michael Jackson was rumoured to be sleeping in an oxygen tank. He wanted to get away from contaminated air and instead breathe clean, stable, undamaged oxygen so it left him looking younger.

In China, people regularly wear masks so they don't breathe in all the toxins in the air, allowing them to counteract the effects on the face and body. They want to stay looking young and avoid damage from everyday chemicals, car fumes and other pollution. You can instantly see the benefits. If you were to do the same daily journey prone to traffic pollution and smog for 25 years, the amount of damage you might inflict on yourself through oxidation would be massive, whereas wearing a mask could potentially increase your lifespan.

People in big cities across the world, including London, already accept this method of protection. If your daily routine means you face pollution, it's worth considering a mask. You may feel odd initially, but you will look even stranger when you hit 45 and your face looks 70 due to pollution.

ALCOHOL

Excessive consumption of alcohol will show in your face as little red blood vessels or spider veins. Small quantities are fine, but too much is dangerous for the liver and heart and makes the face look flushed and sore.

Drinking too much precipitates acne rosacea, dehydrates the skin and deprives it of B vitamins – in particular B12, which aggravates eczema and psoriasis. The sugars in alcohol cause wrinkles and damage skin cells, too. Furthermore, it can be a mood depressant and disrupts sleep, so interrupting night-time repair processes.

EXPRESSION LINES

It may seem like a natural facial movement, but expression lines are habits that we perform voluntarily which can cause deep lines and facial wrinkles in the future.

Every time we adopt an expression line such as furrowing the forehead – say, raising both eyebrows in excitement – a groove forms in the skin. The skin springs back into shape as wrinkles are mobile and temporary when you are younger, but, when skin collagen and elasticity levels deplete through ageing, the lines become permanent as the skin cannot spring back. So you can predict how your face will look when you are older if you look in the mirror and view the expressions you make daily when smiling, talking and even relaxing. When skin loses its agility, these lines can become part of your face profile. Do you like what you see in the mirror? If not, learn to relax the harsh expressions.

SLEEP

Regular sleep is great for the body as it releases Growth Hormone and melatonin and helps fight ageing. If you neglect sleep, this will impact on you mentally, plus your face will show telltale signs, such as bags under the eyes, crow's feet, a tired complexion and saggy skin.

Sleeping with your face buried in a pillow can cause creases. You will notice these on waking as lines in places where you may not even normally make expressions, such as the cheeks or sides of the eyes. This is the result of the face being heavily indented by the weight of the pillow. The best sleeping position is to have the back of your head and neck on one pillow. Duck or goose down pillows are best, and pillow cases in silk or satin will minimise the possibility of pillow lines.

The skin heals and goes back to normal in youth, but as we age the crinkles become deeper and last longer until eventually they are constantly present. This again is down to the skin not having the flexibility to bounce back into shape as the collagen and elastin fibres are no longer so effective.

Try to be aware of your sleep pattern and the way you lie on your pillow. Train yourself to sleep on your back, not your side or front.

STRESS

Anxiety and stress release cortisol into your body and set in motion a cascade of ageing reactions that affect the body and skin. For example, expression lines such as forehead glabellar lines from frowning can become a permanent part of your profile. Try to stop these expressive movements or the damage will eventually become permanent.

Continue, and you will start to experience…

- **Wrinkles on your face:** The years and type of damage will determine the depth and extent of wrinkles. More commonly, they appear around the eyes and mouth, but can surface on the cheeks, above the lips and on the forehead.

- **Sagging skin** through loss of collagen and elasticity: the face begins to droop, particularly around the jaw line and cheeks. Muscles in the skin start to diminish and you're left with a face that shows all the signs of ageing.

- **Turkey neck:** A telltale sign of ageing that is often neglected, resulting in skin thinning and a baggy, creased-looking neck.

- **Eyebags:** The area around the eyes is normally one of the first places to reveal age damage as the skin here is so thin that it holds little collagen and elastin. Lines at the outer corners appear as fine lines and crow's feet, often most visible when you smile or laugh. The upper lids begin to drop and you lose that wide-eyed appearance of youth. Another big concern is bags and dark circles under the eyes.

- **Age spots** normally become visible on those aged 40+ and are usually caused by sun damage over many years.

- **Dryness** as the skin's outer protective oily barrier loses lubrication by evaporation, becoming dehydrated. This combination of dehydrated and dry skin (xerosis) worsens with age, making the skin more brittle, rough and scaly.

Ageing inside and outside the body must be effectively addressed to fix crow's feet, expression lines (forehead furrows, glabellar and nasolabial lines), hollow cheekbones, limp facial muscles, thinning skin, fine lines and deep wrinkles. Getting older on the inside is somewhat predetermined by the gene pool passed down by your family, but a lot is down to you. These issues are addressed in other parts of this book, such as the exercise and nutrition plans, which can alter the inner workings of the body and influence the change in your DNA. Skincare won't actually affect intrinsic ageing, but only complement it.

Ageing on the outside is caused daily by environmental factors such as pollution, ultraviolet rays, smoking, diet, skincare, alcohol, coffee and exercise. It can, however, be controlled and even reversed. This is important as genetics may only account for about 20 per cent of ageing, so we ourselves can control up to 80 per cent. Imagine the changes your face might experience! Dr Nirdosh's Anti-Ageing Skincare Plan will show you how to tackle this.

The skin has two layers: the outer one is called the epidermal layer and the inner layer is the dermis. My skincare plan targets the outer layer for direct treatment. We will treat the inner layer in the next chapter with the Dr Nirdosh Anti-Ageing Supplements Plan.

The outer layer acts as a barrier, preventing foreign particles like water from entering the body. When you take a bath, the water does not go straight through your skin due to the protective mechanism of the epidermis. Skin is normally fed from the inside, heavily relying on the inner layer to feed it with the essential nutrients it needs. The epidermal layer keeps moisture in the skin and prevents it from being lost. I cannot stress enough the importance of this layer as it helps humans to survive and, if damaged, can lead to disaster. Such cases occur in skin burning, where this layer is destroyed with the consequence of evaporative water loss that can be so severe that it might even lead to death.

There are many components to the epidermis and they do amazing things to enhance beauty:

- **Oils** lubricate the skin and reach the outer layer from tiny holes called pores. Once there, they fight off unwanted invaders and stop moisture loss from the skin. Too much stripping of these oily lipids through harsh soaps or sun exposure increases the presence of ulceration, wounds and skin infections.
- **Melanocyte cells** found in the epidermis layer produce melanin, the pigment that gives skin its colour and absorbs ultraviolet rays. The potential for UVA and UVB rays to cause destruction is immense, but melanin helps prevent sunburn. Melanocytes decrease by about 10 to 30 per cent for each decade we live, so our defences to UV radiation weaken, and antioxidants and sun protection become ever more important. With this decline, there is not just a higher risk of wrinkles but also of skin cancer.
- **Langerhans Cells** help to overcome infections and skin inflammation, counteracting excess inflammatory reactions such as psoriasis or dermatitis. They diminish with age and make skin prone to irritation and infectious breakouts.
- **Synthesis of vitamin D** takes place in the epidermis and is induced by UV rays. This vitamin is necessary for bone formation. Deficiency leads to weak bones, even rickets in some extreme cases.

Maintaining a healthy epidermal layer gives your face a natural beauty defence system. You must work hard to keep the skin at its optimum level so that youth and beauty are not compromised; that way, your face can defy ageing.

The inner layer – the dermis – controls temperature and sensory feelings such as touch, pain, sweating and itching. More importantly, it houses collagen, the structural protein that gives skin its firmness.

Elastin fibres lie in the dermis and provide skin with bounce so that, when stretched, it will rapidly return to its original condition. Skin blood supply, nutrients, sweat, oil and hair follicles are also found here. This layer can determine the condition of your face and unlock its beauty but it must be treated from the inside by using the Dr Nirdosh Anti-Ageing Supplements Plan. You'll learn all about this in the next chapter.

A bridge between the two skin layers is called the epidermal dermal junction (EDJ). This has a two-way flow, providing essential nutrients to the outer layer from the inner one (and vice versa), allowing waste products to be discharged, as seen opposite.

You can see from the diagram that both these layers must be treated at the same time to ensure they maintain youth in skin and avoid factors that lead to outward ageing, such as jowls, droopy eyelids, bags under the eyes, skin thinning and wrinkles.

The junction corrodes with age. It is part of the dermis layer so you must never neglect it. Once gone, the rate at which your skin starts to age accelerates as the epidermis begins to break away and lose contact with the dermis. To prevent your delicate epidermal skin layer from withering away, you must take action today. It's

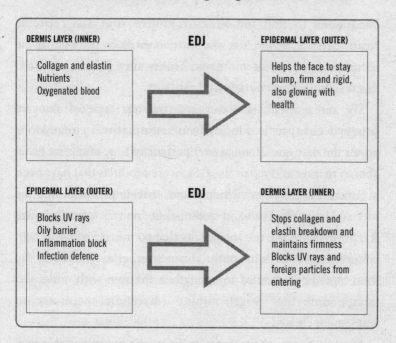

never too late, and the earlier you start, the longer you will hold your natural beauty.

Some of you may think that your skin is beyond repair, but not on my plan! You are about to get the blueprint on how to treat your skin, enabling it to heal its wounds as your face is softened, uplifted and made to look younger. So, what will ensure proper prevention and help age-tarnished skin back to youth? The answer is the powers of a good age-reversing skin treatment that will protect the epidermal layer.

The plan is scientifically designed to give you the treatment necessary for youth. It has been formulated to relieve different types of skin profiles and ages, so you don't need to do all the hard work to find out how to protect your face. Specific treatments will help return your face to youth by prolonging the lifespan of your epidermal layer. This in turn helps protect the dermis, preserving collagen and elasticity.

We are not talking about applying any type of skincare products but specific skincare treatments that will progressively repair the damage sustained over periods of time and force facial skin to recover and repair itself. Skincare products that have been around for many years include creams that simply moisturise the face and help it feel soft and smooth, but don't specifically de-age it. However, we will use treatments that go much further to help restore the face back to youth. This new generation contains the vital ingredients needed to strengthen the skin with molecular components that target minute corrections necessary to implement change.

Most of us use a basic facial moisturising cream and this may have led to an eye cream. On my plan we go beyond this. To give an example, let's look at two other treatments and you can decide which one you would choose:

- **Basic face cream** containing cocoa butter, shea butter and aloe vera *or*
- **Anti-ageing face cream** with collagen, amino acids, high-strength vitamins A, C and E, omega 3, retinol and antioxidants.

You can clearly see that one cream is far superior to the other. The basic cream is made to moisturise the skin but will achieve little else, while the anti-ageing cream is a treatment product. This potent formulation developed to anti-age the face treats the epidermal layer and replenishes lost nutrients and protection. It contains ingredients that help to relax facial expression lines, stimulate collagen production, soften fine lines, plump up the skin and reduce the appearance of wrinkles.

Prolonged use will encourage the skin to become softer, wrinkle-free and uplifted. This can be achieved by feeding the epidermis what it needs, preserving skin collagen levels, protecting the EDJ and the dermis layer. Your face can look decades younger.

This new advanced treatment is not just a face cream, but extends to eye creams, toners and cleansers – all enhanced to become face treatments. You also have a potent new product in the mix: a skin-treatment serum.

Serums are a clever addition to the whole skincare plan because they have capabilities that ordinary creams cannot reach. They allow deeper penetration than face creams alone and contain more powerful ingredients.

THE PLAN

I have spent years medically designing my exclusive anti-ageing skin treatments which provide hundreds of anti-ageing products for head to toe. See www.drnirdosh.com for skincare and supplements product information.

On the Dr Nirdosh Anti-Ageing Skincare Plan, the treatments are precisely targeted and we use products depending on your skin's age. If you are in the mature category, for example, a key concern will be deep wrinkles. Your treatment plan therefore will be geared around addressing these to minimise and soften them, thereby helping you to look younger.

Regardless of skin type, the plan is a five-step regime that requires you to use the following products twice daily in the order set out below:

- **Anti-Ageing Cleanser:** This will be used in the mornings and at night. The aim is to wipe away ageing skin contaminants on the skin's surface, which clog and damage it.

- **Anti-Ageing Toner:** The toner removes excess cleanser residue and then works to tone the skin, preparing it to take your next treatment.

- **Anti-Ageing Serum:** This step is special. The serum is one of the only products to penetrate deep into the skin to enhance protection of the dermis layer via the EDJ. It does this because on the plan we don't use just any serum, we focus on lipid serums. Lipid, oil-based serums are the most effective for deep penetration and skin lubrication. If the serum is comparable to medicated ointments that are oil-based products, it has the ability to penetrate further into the skin, just as oily ointments do, so ingredients have a better chance of cross-exchange between the epidermis and dermis via the EDJ. The serum helps preserve collagen- and elastin-production sources, which in turn help the skin remain taut and plumper for longer. Skin is age-protected during the day and recovers during sleep at night.

- **Eye Cream:** The eyes are the first place to reveal ageing. A dedicated eye treatment that addresses the vast range of eye concerns including bags, fine lines, crow's feet and the like is very important. Depending on your age and skin type, you need the correct eye treatment. For example, if your eyes are only just starting to show the first signs of ageing, then it's essential that you do not miss the opportunity to use eye treatments for this problem. The more appropriately you treat the eye area, the less likely it is that your eyes will suddenly start to age prematurely. Once ageing has occurred, you have to work long and hard to reverse the signs.

- **Face Cream:** Last on the list is the most important treatment and it's essential because the nutrients and molecules contained within it help protect the outside layer. It should last all day and potentially block harsh ageing elements. Such a cream, with the right science, can target fine lines, diminish wrinkles, heal rashes and block sun rays and age damage. It can help new collagen synthesis and turn dull, dry skin into a brighter, hydrated, smoother complexion. But more than all this, it allows a time-damaged face to become much more youthful.

  This is a really important treatment because the face treatment cream gives you all the results in one. If you miss out on this, or rarely use a face treatment cream then you really are setting yourself up to become a victim of premature ageing. Leaving it too late can mean you may have to rectify the damage later, which will be a more demanding and time-consuming task.

You may normally spend only a minute on your daily skincare routine, but this must change as we are now treating the skin with a prescribed plan. Your skin will progressively repair and even reverse some of the age damage. My treatment plan takes 8–10 minutes, morning and night, and you need to allow for that amount of time to achieve the desired results. Apply each treatment like this:

1. Using a cotton pad, apply the anti-ageing cleanser to the entire face and neck, especially regions covered in make-up and oil-prone areas such as the nose and forehead.

2. With fresh cotton pads, gently apply pressure to remove grime and cleanse the face and neck using upward and outward strokes. Do not pull the skin too harshly and be extremely gentle around the eyes and cheeks.

3. Once the face is cleansed, move on to the toner – this process should take between 30 seconds and a minute. If the toner has a spray action, it can be sprayed directly on to the face, avoiding the delicate eye region. Using cotton pads, thoroughly remove any cleanser residue and remaining impurities and then pat the skin all over with cotton pads to enhance the toning effect. If there is no spray action, dispense the toner directly on to cotton pads.

4. The skin is now ready for the serum. Dispense this on to your fingertips and, with a light, circular massage action, apply evenly to the face. Concentrate heavier doses and longer massaging action over lines, wrinkles and areas of age damage – you want maximal absorption through the open pores to

reduce the appearance of lines and flow towards the dermis and EDJ. Stay clear of the eye area: the ingredients in serums are too strong for this and may result in sore puffy eyes.

5. When you have finished the whole face, continue with the neck regions. With serums, do not neglect the neck – it is part of the application process that works to tighten and reduce ageing concerns, such as turkey neck. Again, this is essential as the lipid oil-based serum has the capability to go deep and work on the whole neck. For the neck, use pressure from both hands: start at the base and work in upward massage strokes from both hands to blend towards the chin. Repeat this stroking action a few times. You must spend a minimum of 60 seconds on the face and, again, the same amount of time massaging the serum deep into the neck.

6. Now, let's move on to the eye region. To apply the eye cream, dispense a pea-sized amount on to one finger and dab small dots of cream along the upper and lower lids. Now, using a light tapping action, blend the cream into the skin, starting at the outer eye corners and working your way towards the inner ones. Repeat for the lower and upper lids, massaging the cream in the opposite direction to crow's feet and creases. Under the eyes, where accumulating fluid causes puffiness, apply a subtle pressing motion, working your way from the outside towards the inner eye zone and extending to about 2cm (1in) below the eyes to cover the whole area. This creates a stimulating action that helps to shift any congestion.

7. By now, the serum should have been absorbed into the skin, so we can apply the face cream. Using your fingers, place small

dots of moisturiser on to the cheeks, upper lip area, chin, forehead, sides of the eyes and neck. With fingertips and a circular massage action, blend the face cream into the skin. Work against gravity in areas of lines and wrinkles. Apply deep pressure in these parts, but don't tug or stretch the skin too harshly. Again, you must never forget the neck. Massage the cream into the whole area using both hands and applying upward strokes. Spend 2–3 minutes massaging moisturiser into the facial and neck skin, as with the serum.

So now you know the application process, we will move on to the next part of the plan, the Skincare Blueprint for your skin profile, addressing those unanswered questions.

WHICH TREATMENTS DO I NEED?

This is a dilemma for everyone and a big factor when it comes to selecting skincare products. Many people give up simply because they don't know which type suits them. My unique plan will become the basis of your morning and evening skincare routine. The great thing is that, as your circumstances change, you just select the next blueprint for your altered skin profile. It has been developed so that all members of the family can be on the plan together. Mothers can follow their scheme, daughters have a treatment and so do men.

The Blueprint

With each decade comes a new change and our physical appearance becomes different as the shape of our faces changes.

Our hair and bone structure alter, too. Knowing this, it's important that the anti-ageing skincare treatment works selectively based on requirements for your skin age. The blueprints that follow are developed for your age and are specific to skin for that age profile.

Twenties

The skin in our twenties is vibrant, young and normally untarnished by ageing, but the external appearance doesn't give a true reflection of the internal workings and the changes developing inside.

It is at this infancy stage that you have the chance to set the path as to how your skin ages and will appear each decade hereafter, so it's essential to look after skin cells and really nurture the epidermal layer. The great thing is that youth is on your side and is still working with you, not against you. Internally, the cells are fast dividing, turnover is good and old cells are equally replaced by healthy new ones. Excellent skin-cell production allows younger, fully formed cells to keep the complexion looking line-free, smooth and glowing with health.

The epidermis is well fed by the dermis layer because the EDJ is intact; the dermis itself is full of an organised array of collagen and elastin, retaining firm tensile strength. All seems well, not a hint of a wrinkle in sight. That's the good news. However, the bad news is that, invisible to the naked eye, the skin suffers the impact of ultraviolet radiation, inflammation, dietary and damaging lifestyle factors only visible through a microscope. This lays the foundations for future damage, slowly harming cell DNA, cell walls, dermal extracellular matrix and the EDJ. Soon it becomes visible as fine lines, which will progress into deep wrinkles. We must prevent this.

Twenties Profile		
SKIN PROBLEM	**WHY**	**SOLUTION**
Adolescence	Sebaceous glands very active in producing sebum to leave the skin oily, with clogged pores, acne, blackheads and whiteheads	Gentle exfoliating washes, antiseptics (tea tree, liquorice, witch hazel, salicylic acid, vitamin C, manuka, nicotinamide, vitamin B5, retinoids)
Oral contraceptive pill	Excess oestrogen and progesterone cause uneven skin, brown pigmentation patches and enhanced sensitivity to sun damage	Vitamin B5 (panthenol), B6, E, C, EFAs, broad-spectrum UV sun protection
Sun exposure	Microscopic inflammation and collagen damage, fine lines plus dry, scaly skin	Antioxidants, ellagic acid, UV sun protection, emollient based creams
Alcohol, smoking, bad diet	Stress-hormone release, dull skin, fine lines, rough and blotchy, sallow skin, dermatitis, acne	Zinc, B vitamins, vitamin C, omega 3, antioxidants, plus skin-brightening agents like fruit extracts

The blueprint shows the skin-ageing issues of skin in its twenties. It affects the dermis and epidermis layers and has the power to accelerate ageing. The symptoms show on the skin's surface and the face so the correct treatments must be used to attack the ageing culprits head-on.

At this age, the hormones in your body are in a yo-yo process. Sebaceous oil glands produce sebum, which leaves the skin oily, clogs pores and encourages acne, blackheads and whiteheads. Left alone, some forms of acne can cause permanent scarring and make your face appear wrinkly. You must use gentle exfoliating face washes, face creams, cleansers and toners that contain antiseptics such as tea tree, liquorice, witch hazel, salicylic acid, vitamin C, nicotinamide, vitamin B5, manuka and retinoids. These will help rebalance the skin and keep sebum under control. The correct skin-sensitive acne treatments will reduce the chances of serious ageing skin concerns, leaving your skin young and protected.

If you are taking contraceptives, then you may be producing excess oestrogen and progesterone. These can cause the dermis to react with the appearance of uneven skin with patches of brown pigmentation. The pill can also make skin more sensitive to sun damage. Tackle this with a face treatment containing vitamins B5, B6, E and C, EFAs and a UV defence to help protect the skin and directly address these concerns.

Sun exposure dramatically speeds up ageing. At this young age, the dermis layer is vulnerable because it has never experienced such damage in the form of microscopic inflammation, collagen damage, fine lines, dry and scaly skin. If you do not treat your face daily, you risk looking decades older and skin continuously exposed in this way will progressively sag.

Treat the skin here with a face cream containing antioxidants, ellagic acid, dark berry fruit extracts such as pomegranate, blueberry, EFAs and UV protection. They provide the skin with antioxidant protectors to help neutralise cell damage and extend skin-cell life.

You can hold on to youth for a long time, but you must avoid the guilty pleasures of excess alcohol, smoking or a bad diet. These choices will start to create ageing habits that you may find it hard to shake off later and will force the secretion of the stress hormones. These occur internally, but also show themselves externally as dull skin, fine lines, rough and blotchy, sallow skin, dermatitis and pimples. Use a vitamin- and mineral-intensified cream containing zinc, B and C vitamins and omega 3. Quickly and effectively, these micronutrients help to heal blemishes and imperfections so your skin won't enter its thirties looking sore and sun-blushed, with a rash-ridden texture.

The products you now select become the blueprint for skin in its twenties and you must remember the following routine: cleanser, toner, serum, eye and face cream. You can change and refine this, but the blueprint is your personal skin doctor and allows you to be precise in selecting anti-ageing treatments for young, tender skin. Choose products that will assist the skin in its twenties correctly and you will enter your thirties allowing others to see your beautiful face has been well preserved.

Thirties

Skin in its thirties is experiencing the first real obvious signs of ageing. The biggest difference to our twenties is that facial features and shape are now stamped out. Your face is fully developed and in its thirties can look most defined. The downside is that, even though you may feel that you have learned to like and accept the way your face looks, the rate at which your body is geared to age is now much faster than in your twenties.

The trick in the thirties blueprint is to slow down the rate of damage, as in this decade the skin will go through drastic changes. Skin-cell turnover slows so that cells are lost faster than they can be replaced. For example, what we need to worry about is Co Enzyme Q10, which is one of the first antioxidants and cell metabolism boosters to leave the body and cause cell production to slow.

The once-dewy, glowing skin of your twenties is now replaced by the first signs of ageing: dull, dry skin and fine age lines; at the same time the vital protein responsible for the frame and definition of the face starts to decay. Collagen and elastin fibres become sloppy and progressive DNA damage causes skin cells to lose vitality.

The skin can become overworked and show the telltale signs in the form of broken capillaries (telangiectasia), age spots (melasma) and acne rosacea. These are common manifestations in our thirties – acne rosacea particularly, which flares with inflammatory red patches, tiny pimples and heightened skin sensitivity. Now your skin is more prone to age damage. Dynamic wrinkles (the mobile ones that happen when we make expressions) can start to become static, permanent lines on the face.

Loss of elasticity means it becomes difficult for the skin to relax fully, even once an expression has disappeared. Do this too often and expression lines become a permanent part of the complexion. Once permanent, they become static wrinkles and are hard to shift.

Women often become pregnant in their thirties so a rush of oestrogen and progesterone affects the skin. Protective and repairing skincare treatments are needed. We must heal existing damage and shield effectively against further ageing.

Thirties Profile		
SKIN PROBLEM	**WHY**	**SOLUTION**
First signs of ageing, including dull skin	Reduced cell turnover, deficiency of co-enzyme Q10	Skin polishing agents and radiance restorers like olive, co-enzyme Q10, vitamin C
Broken capillaries, acne rosacea, tiny pimples, age spots/freckles, melasma	Inflammation, hormonal/pregnancy induced skin changes	Antioxidants, vitamin C, retinoids, B vitamins, zinc
Dry and dehydrated skin	Deficiency of lipids and water	EFAs (Essential Fatty Acids), avocado, omega 3, 6 and 9, vitamin E, hyaluronic preservers, NFF complex
Dynamic wrinkles, fine lines, especially around the eyes and dark circles, perioral lines (lines around lips), nasolabial lines (smile lines running from the corners of the nose to the corners of the mouth)	Early onset damage to collagen, elastin begins to lose recoil, expression lines deepen	Antioxidant protectors, collagen preservers, UV blockers, green tea, EGCG, vitamin C, vitamin E, centella asciatica, resveratrol, vitamin K for eyes

This is a critical stage because you start to see age signs and must therefore introduce damage control. A lot of the damage is harm to skin collagen, elastin and co-enzyme Q10 loss, so the skin must be replenished, repaired and protected.

A deficiency of co-enzyme Q10 will show in the skin's surface, starting the process of early skin-cell death. It is essential that all skincare-treatment plans in your thirties have sufficient metabolic stimulators. Combine with skin-polishing olive OPCs (Oligomeric Proanthocyanidin) and vitamin C on the face to counteract epidermal harm.

The skin's capability to hold water decreases, which causes it to be seriously dehydrated, so elevating the first signs of ageing. This is not just restricted to water, but also fats (lipids) in the skin. You must take action with a range of skin treatments that contain some form of EFAs. Avocado, omega 3, 6 and 9, vitamin E and hyaluronic acid preservers such as NFF complex will all keep skin lubricated, reducing the possibility of dry, flaky skin, which can rapidly progress to age lines.

Dynamic (non-permanent) lines will be a worse problem. We don't consciously control the way we make expressions like smiling, but the outcome of consistent, habitual facial emotions can enforce permanent face lines. These result in fine lines, especially around the eyes, leading to deep lines that can spread all over the face as you smile. There may be dark circles under the eyes and smile lines around the lips and from the corners of the nose to the corners of the mouth.

Skin becoming less tactile is an early symptom of loss of collagen and elastin. The damage has already been done in the dermis layer and is now spreading outwards to the skin's surface. The result is that your outer epidermal layer is now weaker. We must address this in the thirties blueprint as one of the most important parts of your skin treatment to protect your face and prevent dynamic lines.

Finally, the skin will receive a personal prescription that allows it to become agile and responsive again. The fixing process will alter the surface, which in turn can help defend the EDJ and the dermis. To treat it, we need to load the face with powerful antioxidant protectors. These will help to stop premature skin-cell breakdown and provide the technology to remain strong and youthful. Powerful antioxidants are green tea EGCGs, vitamins C and E and resveratrol. They act as collagen preservers and also shield against environmental pollution.

UV blockers when exposed to the sun must be an integral part of your thirties skincare treatment as the rays will damage the skin's collagen and structure. Finally, you must use eye-treatment creams with all the antioxidants and EFAs, plus vitamin K. This is essential to ease sluggish blood flow under the eyes. Following this blueprint in your thirties allows you to experience younger, stronger skin into your forties.

The Dr Nirdosh treatments are prescribed to a range of celebrities as they contain all the molecular components needed for your skin blueprint and are tailor-made for your specific age profile.

Forties

Skin in its forties is about to experience a rollercoaster ride and below is the blueprint to fight back successfully. Celebrities in their forties who have defied this decade well include *Sex and the City* star Sarah Jessica Parker and fellow actress Liz Hurley, who is also a clothes designer. More serious issues challenge the face now and make it age much more rapidly. We must do all we can to halt this process.

The most dangerous cause of ageing in your forties is when the dermis and epidermal layer begin to separate. At this stage, the EDJ starts to split so the dermis and epidermis lose contact, which means the skin cannot properly exchange the nutrients and substances necessary for repair. The internal damage will already have set in to leave the outer epidermal layer weakened and worn out.

Further factors that also determine your skin condition include the amount of exercise you may have done. If this is very little, then your skin may be loose and show early signs of sagging through facial-muscle loss.

Facial-muscle loss, dermal thinning and falling levels of the sex hormones oestrogen and testosterone leave behind remnants of a haggard face. Skin in its forties naturally becomes thinner and drier, while the soft expression lines of your thirties now become deep indentations.

The skin around the eyes becomes fragile and crow's feet extend further. Eyelids start to droop and the under-eye area becomes puffy, with accumulating fluid and dark circles setting up home. The skin enters a pre-menopausal state and already incurs a huge loss of anti-ageing hormones. This loss may induce the body into an acceptance that it is becoming old, but my anti-ageing skincare plan will fight back.

Skin in its forties must incorporate augmenting protein to boost Growth Hormone and enhance your oestrogen levels. If neglected in the pre-menopausal days, your skin will become dull and washed out, but it does not have to be like that.

Collagen destruction is rising, causing the skin to quickly lose its stability, and elastin fibres become stiff. Deep grooves begin to line the face and brown hyperpigmentation patches become ever more evident. The skin needs relaxants such as boswellia to calm and heal expression lines, as well as collagen revivers, multivitamin complexes, especially A, C and E, zinc and elasticity preservers such as kalpariane algae.

Ensure skincare products are rich in hyaluronate elevators such as NFF and glucosamine, which help to hold moisture as evaporative water loss increases and enhances facial lines. Skincare must be rich in lipids such as omega 3 and 6 to restore diminishing sebum levels so the surface is always well lubricated.

The face will look more angular, while the jaw line appears flaccid and less distinct. Skincare must be geared towards plumping up and replacing nutrients so wrinkles and age scars are minimised. The skin needs to be fully prepared to tackle menopause hormonal losses due in the next decade. If your skin is weak in its forties, it stands no chance of withstanding ageing in its fifties.

You must exert intense effort in applying skincare and using the right massage techniques to help stimulate skin toning and lifting. The face needs all the attention you can give it and a corrective array of pre-menopausal ingredients to reinstate a youthful complexion.

If you have spent your youth basking in the sun, then solar elastosis (amorphous clumps of elastin) will have left big creases on the face and they will cause havoc on surrounding collagen fibres, pushing them out of the way and ruining their orderly structure. Unattended eyes will show full-blown age damage and need specific eye-region smoothing and rectifying ingredients such as eyebright, vitamins A, C, E and K, as well as collagen and elasticity reinforcers.

Forties Profile		
SKIN PROBLEM	**WHY**	**SOLUTION**
Deep-set static (permanent) wrinkles and crow's feet, loss of firmness starts to show, spider veins, enlarged pores, puffy darkening eye zone	Collagen degradation and insufficient reproduction of sebum as sebaceous glands lose function, dermis of eye thins	Collagen revivers, minerals, expression line relaxants – boswellia, vitamins A, C and E, B vitamins, zinc, antioxidants, plus vitamin K for eyes
Skin sags, drooping, hollow cheeks begin to show	Elasticity declines and solar elastosis (thick, immobile skin creases) from previous sun exposure	Elasticity preservers like kalpariane algae, vitamins A, C and E
Rough and dry, dehydrated skin	Dead skin cells pile up and cell turnover goes down, loss of glycosaminoglycans (GAGs), especially hyaluronic acid levels; sebum (oil) production declines, trans-epidermal water loss accelerates	Hyaluronic acid boosters, sebum, restorers, EFAs, omega 3 and 6, hydration enhancers, NFF, hyaluronic acid, glucosamine, lipid serums vital
Dermal thinning, pre-menopausal state skin, hyperpigmentation	Decreased sex hormones (oestrogen and testosterone), decreased Growth Hormone, decreased amino acids and protein production declines	Extracellular matrix plumpers, collagen molecules, protein and amino acid complexes

Fifties

A lot of the natural skin protectors disappear in our fifties. Collagen and elasticity levels quickly deplete to leave the skin looking slack and old, knocking our confidence. Signs such as smokers' lines around the lips become more defined and now settle permanently. The skin may have lost its ability to spring back and expression lines are carved into the face as everlasting wrinkles.

The skin appears much thinner, almost translucent. As the EDJ continues to break away, so blood supply to the epidermis and nutrient exchange is vastly reduced. Skin will find it harder to produce and retain oils and trans-epidermal water loss increases, making it look crispy and dehydrated. This leaves a flaky, crumpled and flaccid complexion, vulnerable to cuts and grazes.

Another big visual difference is that the face will have visible pigment changes. The skin becomes far duller and greyer, losing its natural healthy colour and vitality. It often shows freckles normally caused by excessive sun tanning.

Menopausal oestrogen depletion and Growth Hormone loss cause demineralisation and change in shape of the cheekbones so they look hollow and fat shifts from beneath facial skin, giving a gaunt appearance. Wrinkles become deeply engraved and the face becomes tarnished with spider veins (broken capillaries), acne rosacea (red patchiness) hyperpigmentation (brown age spots) and widening skin pores.

The jawbone becomes covered in droopy skin and its definition disappears as the jowls take over. Serious loss of muscle, collagen and elastin has taken place and left behind an aged-looking face. Yet such people as Madonna escape the worst of these symptoms. Again, I cannot stress too much the importance of a really effective anti-ageing treatment plan. Skincare must be dedicated to mature skin; with toning, lifting, cell metabolism boosting and retexturing action for a smoother, more even skin surface. New, healthy skin is needed to come through and repair all that outside destruction. The right treatment includes high-strength vitamins, minerals, strong antioxidants and oestrogen-mimicking substances.

Fifties Profile		
SKIN PROBLEM	**WHY**	**SOLUTION**
Permanent wrinkles, expression lines set deep, jowls, drooping eyelids, xerosis (dry skin) increases, turkey neck evolves	Chronic dermal damage, breakdown of elastin, dehydration as GAGs go down, sebum production declines so the skin's oily lubrication becomes depleted, TEWL continues to elevate, neck loses rigidity and becomes flaccid from collagen and elastin loss	Emollient/ointment-based products high in lipids, rosehip, retinol, collagen boosters, folic acid; elasticity promoters: kalpariane algae, other seaweed and yeast extracts, amino acids, boswellia
Skin infections and age invaders make their way in more easily	Loss of Langerhans cells weakens skin defences and healing powers, skin-repair ability drops, loss of copper peptides makes repair a difficult task	Copper, vitamin complexes, especially A, C and E; antioxidants such as selenium, superoxide dismutase
Patchy skin, age spots, open pores, thinned skin	Menopausal loss of oestrogen and progesterone massively impacts skin, loss of anti-ageing hormones and protein synthesis continues to increase	Soya peptides, yam extracts, soybean, ginkgo biloba
Sluggish and grey, bumpy skin; epidermis blisters, grazes and cracks	Slowed cell metabolism, static lymphatic system leaves toxins, vitamin D production declines, blood supply goes down, EDJ splits – lost nutrients and oxygenated blood to epidermis as it loses connection with dermis	Vitamin D, zinc, B vitamins and vitamin E

Dermal supporters are needed to conserve moisture due to excessive TEWL. Lipid-rich skincare products with emollient action can be absorbed deeply and release their goodness, while combating extremely dry skin. Cell membranes need EFAs and treatments for mature skin must be applied twice daily without fail.

Adhere as strictly as you can to the Dr Nirdosh Anti-Ageing Skincare Plan. To counteract permanent wrinkles, expression lines, jowls and drooping eyelids, skincare must be high in oils and ingredients such as rosehip, retinol, collagen boosters, folic acid, amino acids and elasticity promoters like kalpariane algae or other seaweed. These will slow the damage and fix the present condition of the skin.

The skin profile is now more vulnerable to infections as the loss of vital cells weakens its immune support and healing powers. At this stage, the ability to repair itself and resist foreign invaders drops drastically. Less vitamin D is produced and the skin is generally lacking across the board in all vitamin and mineral complexes.

Use creams with collagen, copper, zinc and vitamin complexes, especially A, C, D and E. Antioxidants such as selenium and superoxide dismutase help fight further cell breakdown. Age spots must be tackled or they will increase further. Skincare containing soya peptides and ginkgo biloba works directly on the spots, spider veins and oestrogen-depleted skin.

Stop tanning if you are still doing so. Protect your skin against the sun's rays by using UV protector and wear sunglasses at every opportunity – the eyes are far more vulnerable than elsewhere on the face. Ignoring this will lead to increasingly deeper wrinkles.

To banish the lifeless, dull grey look, treatments should be equipped in a strengthening way. This is the best method to restore a healthy youthful radiance, provide a shield from ageing and mend skin wounds. If you have not done so already, give up cigarettes and cut back on alcohol. They harm your skin, making you look older.

Heighten Growth Hormone levels by using the exercise plan (see Chapter 5) and enhance skin immunity with nutritional power. Foods rich in protein, beta-carotene and a range of vitamins will help repair wrinkles.

Women Over 60

The beauty of stars in their sixties shines on: Raquel Welch, Susan Sarandon, Sigourney Weaver, Dame Helen Mirren, Goldie Hawn, Mia Farrow and Grace Jones are all stunning. And so are you, if you look after your skin. These women care for their skin every day with anti-ageing treatments. Your skin will have aged, too, but there are lots of things you can do to keep it attractive.

The choice is yours: you can simply give up or be stunning like the new Cougar women on the prowl for men half their age. Yes, they really do exist and they do marry younger men! Joan Collins is happily married to one, as are half the women mentioned above.

So the sixties is not an age of dismay for your skin, but a time of liberation and reinvention in which you unveil a new, more experienced, more confident you – learning to love the skin you're in. The skin will appear with profound folds and lines in regions you didn't anticipate; it won't be as tactile as it once was. Its ability to absorb vitamins will be reduced, delaying wound repairs and there will be no hiding from liver spots (lentigines), skin tags, warts and cherry angiomas (blood spots).

Cutaneous neoplasms (skin cancers) also pose a real threat

now, so any suspicious moles or other dubious skin alterations need investigation. The epidermal junction has now moved a long way apart from the dermis, making healing and communication between the two skin layers extremely difficult.

If you have smoked all your life, the chances are your skin will look a decade or two older than 60, as the smoking-induced destruction of elasticity – nicotinic elastosis – has taken effect with thick creases of skin folding over one another. If you're still a sun goddess, further elasticity breakdown will occur as severe wrinkling and wilting take their toll.

The body will encounter a severe loss of anti-ageing hormones, with Growth Hormone, oestrogen and testosterone dwindling. So the skin becomes coarse, covered in grooves and follows suit of the rest of the body, as everything sags south.

Hair grows in odd regions such as the chin, ears and nose. The skin becomes more delicate, readily tearing, bruising and scarring. Also, the eyes squint as everything closes in around the eye orbits. Skin here will be particularly thin and brittle.

Skin pallor is common, resulting in a lack of nutrient-fresh oxygenated blood. Nerves lose their high-performance ability so sensation control becomes a problem – temperature, pain and even pleasure sensations become harder to detect. This exposes us to injury as withdrawal reflexes become sluggish. The emaciated, leaky nature of the skin, combined with a lowering of its immune defences, allows damaging elements to force their way in easily and cause infections, inflammation and a breakdown of composition. But do not despair: much of this can be addressed, healed and some damage even reversed.

The Dr Nirdosh Anti-Ageing Skincare Plan

Sixties Profile		
SKIN PROBLEM	**WHY**	**SOLUTION**
Deep skin wrinkles, saggy fragile skin, pale in colour, and lost skin sensitivity; jowls take over and skin becomes limp all over, eyes become hollow and squinted. Eyebrows and eyelids drop, dark circles and bags are pronounced, eye skin particularly delicate and tears readily	Collagen and elasticity lost, thermoregulation becomes impaired and nerves are not so good at sensing pain, touch or movement; lost sensory perception increases the risk of skin injury; vascularity is lost, plus the emaciated, leaky nature of mature skin makes it vulnerable to fast-paced ageing attack	Tighten limp skin, especially jowls and neck, with collagen, skin firmers and elasticity boosters; EFAs vitamin A/retinol, skin-cell immunity boosters – vitamin C and antioxidants, hydrolysed proteins, amino acids, magnesium, zinc, vitamin E tocotrienols
Complexion has liver spots (lentigines), skin tags, warts and cherry angiomas (blood spots); cutaneous neoplasms cause danger, skin infections and inflammation occurs	Decreased ability to absorb essential minerals like zinc, iron and other vitamins delays wound repair. EDJ becomes flatter and moves further apart; skin-cell immunity is weak, therefore infections and foreign contaminants can enter	Mineral complexes, vitamins A, C and D, antioxidants, zinc, calcium, kojic acid, allantoin, UVA and UVB protection; keep eyes covered with UV-protective shades
Nicotonic elastosis – skin become leathery and crumpled; also coarse. The face is covered in grooves, plus hair growth occurs in odd regions like the chin, ears and nasal areas	Smoking-induced elasticity destruction now adds years to an ageing face; severe loss of anti-ageing hormones –oestrogen, testosterone and Growth Hormone – advances the look of old, haggard skin	Mild exfoliating wash to remove rough skin and dead cells; elasticity strengtheners – marine/yeast/algae extracts, vitamins C and E, soya, yam, iron/folic acid, biotin, nicotinamide, panthenol
Rough skin patches, plus severe dryness (xerosis) all over; cheekbones become hollow and thin, elongated features	Hyperkeratosis causes dead skin cells to clump together, bones become thin and demineralised, plus subcutaneous fat shifts from beneath the facial skin, making it even thinner	Toning, lifting, boosting new healthy skin-cell production; repair surface damage with high-strength vitamins, minerals and dermal supporters. Lipid-rich skincare, emollients/ointments that can be deeply absorbed, ceramides, GLA (omega 6), borage seed, lecithin, and glycolic acid

A very strict anti-ageing plan must be followed daily as a vital part of cell rehabilitation. Supplements, nutrition and exercises are needed to reinject declining hormonal activity. We need to rid the skin of hyperkeratosis (dead skin cells clumped together which give skin a rough, bumpy texture) and renew the surface, while tightening limp muscle tissue so the face appears naturally lifted. This will also help strengthen elasticity and collagen fibres, while tautening dragging jowls.

Pronounced dryness (xerosis) compounds wrinkles and makes the skin look shrivelled. Use an ointment or emollient cream rich in vital sebum-replacing oil-based lubrication to treat this dryness and halt accelerated evaporative water loss.

A firmer, younger-looking, resurfaced complexion will need collagen and Growth Hormone enhancers, skin firmers, marine/yeast/algae elasticity strengtheners, plus EFAs, GLA omega 6, ceramides, lecithin, vitamin A/retinol, skin-cell immunity boosters (vitamins C and E and antioxidants), hydrolysed proteins, amino acids, magnesium, zinc, vitamin E tocotrienols, calcium, soya peptides, yam extracts, iron/folic acid, biotin, nicotinamide and panthenol.

Men's Skin

A man's skin has a totally different composition from a woman's – it needs another combination of nutrients to correct cell turnover, guard against wrinkles and make repairs. Men have a thicker dermis layer that holds more collagen and elastin fibres. To maintain rigidity and firmness, the skin must be provided with substances such as collagen, proteins, echium or silica that can penetrate to the required depths. Male skin also has a thicker epidermis layer, which results in the accumulation of dead surface cells and a dull, tired-looking complexion. To overcome this, it needs replenishment with precise antioxidant fortification such as OPCs and skin-regenerating vitamin A or retinol molecules.

The heavy density of hair follicles and sebaceous glands can lead to excessive sebum production and acne breakouts, so zinc oxide and vitamins C and E are all vital to help keep metabolic processes regulated and skin in an anti-inflammatory state.

Men's body formation relies on stable levels of testosterone: a critical, male-dominating, anti-ageing hormone, whose levels rapidly decline with age. Boosting internal supplies with Testoster-Force tablets, a specialist formula for men, will raise stamina, strength and libido, and helps prevent osteoporosis, lean-tissue deterioration and organ disease.

Using dedicated skincare for men has vast benefits: specific moisturisers supply the skin with specialist repair and recovery components to allow you to wake up with younger-looking skin.

Chapter 8

The Dr Nirdosh Anti-Ageing Supplements Plan

THERE IS A misconception that cosmetic surgery brings back the youthful looks of both sexes. Actually, these serious operations are just a short-term fix that requires topping up when the results fail.

Many celebrities used to have a little bit of surgery here and there, but they ended up with that expressionless, wind-tunnel look. Now that has all changed.

Why the U-turn? Surgery does nothing to stop ageing processes. In fact, as the years go by, people age far faster so the surgery turns out to be useless. A lot of stars fear it is ruining their faces for the long term, too. If this development has caused many celebrities to say no to the knife, what secret methods are they now using instead to stop ageing? My clients feel they cannot live without my daily cosmetic youth pills – anti-ageing supplements that help prolong their youthful looks and make them live longer.

Ageing occurs from within but shows externally so we must

treat the internal ageing directly, otherwise the body will go on ageing, with the damage showing on our faces and all over our bodies. Treatment with my daily anti-ageing supplements heals and even reverses the damage. I prescribe them to my celebrity clients and now you too can share their secrets.

The goal is to tackle age damage head-on and to treat the core of the problem with the power of the supplements. When you feed the body correctly, you replenish internal losses of specific micronutrients and age-defying substances so the body puts a brake on ageing from within, allowing you to look younger, sexier and healthier.

Minuscule doses make an incredibly big difference, helping to optimise and complete reactions in the body. Medically, supplements have proved lifesavers for those suffering from serious debilitating diseases where nutrition is restricted. Parenteral nutrition, where liquid food and supplementation is inserted through a gastro-intestinal tube, is commonly used in hospitals to feed those unable to ingest by mouth.

With supplements, the body receives tiny amounts of essential micronutrients – vitamins, minerals, trace elements, antioxidants and EFAs – that can easily be missed out on during the day, even though they may only be required in amounts of less than 100mg. They have an extraordinary ability to slow ageing and help people live longer.

Even in developed countries such as Britain and the US, where food is available in vast quantities compared with the amount available in developing nations, malnutrition is still common. It fast-forwards ageing and is a pathological condition caused by:

- Insufficient micronutrients: vitamins, co-factors, micronutrients and other trace elements
- A lack of sufficient calories and too few essential micronutrients.

OBESITY AND OVEREATING

Certain micronutrients are vital for metabolic functioning so that the body cannot complete tasks without them. You might be eating plenty of food, but, if it's the wrong stuff, then poor nutrition can cause ill health and premature ageing.

What we need daily is not stacks of any kind of nutrition, but stacks of quality, anti-ageing food. It's difficult to meet our requirements from high-street cafés or stale supermarket sandwiches. Yet for most of us to pre-prepare every meal before heading off to work is living in fairytale land, so, as well as being careful to pick up the right foods on the go, a daily dose of supplements is a fine way to ensure you don't miss out on essential micronutrients that the body cannot make for itself.

Malnutrition does not just affect those who don't, or can't, eat enough. In an ironic health backlash, Western countries have created a problem with overeating and obesity. The junk-food epidemic has caused a malnutrition outbreak. Unbalanced quantities of macronutrients (carbohydrates, fats and protein) and micronutrients shackle physical condition and cost the NHS and similar bodies a fortune to rectify.

The World Health Organisation (WHO) is tackling micronutrient-related epidemics, especially in developing countries, where they know action could save up to a billion lives.

The right nutrition can have such an influence on lengthening people's lives that by 2025 it is forecast that there will be 1.2 billion over-60s living in the world and 2.5 billion by 2050, 75 per cent of them in developed countries.

If your body doesn't receive the right amounts of vitamins or minerals, it will not be able to perform optimally and its own repairs will be in jeopardy. To meet all those needs through food gets harder as we become older and our bodies cannot process nutrients from food quite so efficiently as they did in our youth. Absorption from the intestine is less good, enzymes are not so active at breaking foods down, nutrient production and conversion starts to fail us, we become nutrient-resistant and our cell receptors lose sensitivity. Taking supplements therefore becomes vital, but how do you know which ones are correct for your skin type, body problem and age?

The Dr Nirdosh Anti-Ageing Supplements Plan does this for you. For the first time you will have a personal regime which allows you to stop trailing through stores with the bewildered look of someone who doesn't know what to buy and leaves with nothing, more confused than when they started.

My daily supplements are the most vital parts of the jigsaw puzzle to help you hold back the decades. Without them, you have to work hard to de-age the body. You need a clear nutritional plan, an effective exercise regime and a dedicated anti-ageing skincare-treatment plan just to have a fighting chance.

If you think surgery is the answer, then you're in for a shock. The internal damage will continue regardless of any operation – no surgeon's knife can stop that. But if you want a face with a noticeable lift and to slow down the signs of ageing, the answer is supplements.

YOUR SECRET WEAPON

Supplements have the extraordinary ability to delay ageing signs and to help you live longer, yet most people do not know about them. If I could give you an anti-ageing pill that is natural and safe, and could help give you a face-lift, would you be interested?

My supplements replenish the body with the vitamins, proteins, hormones and antioxidants that are slowly lost with age. None of the other anti-ageing disciplines mentioned in this book is as simple as taking a single tablet to get results. To give you an example, a protein essential to prevent the face from sagging is collagen. We can now take an age-specific, collagen-enhancing supplement to help fight its internal loss. The body uses the ingredients it contains to help synthesise new proteins and develop fresh, healthy collagen. Prolonged use can promote a plumper, smoother face. That's why supplements are your secret weapon against ageing.

Remember, my supplements plan is safe, effective and essential because many nutrients cannot be manufactured inside the body so we must turn to capsules and tablets. The trick is to take the right ones at the right time, if you want results.

WHY YOUTH PILLS WORK

Beautiful Parisians don't get fat or unattractive with time – they have discovered the massive benefits of supplements and consider them the fountain of youth. They use them in their daily skin and body plans.

Manufacturers have been targeting continental Europe for years with anti-ageing skin and body supplements – and with great success. They have been known to outsell skin creams. Why? Because European women know they work by treating the source of the problem – the internal skin layer or dermis – dramatically reducing the facial signs of ageing. They see face creams as a secondary double protection, not the first point of action.

When skin shows signs of ageing, it is usually due to damage from the dermis. Lines, wrinkles and sagging then reveal themselves on the outer layer, the epidermis. You can treat the epidermis with anti-ageing treatment creams, but to reach the dermis you need supplements that can tackle this layer.

It makes more sense to prevent the damage in the first place so you don't have to treat it. Daily anti-ageing pills will repair and protect the dermis. Indeed, the power of supplements can alter the rate of external facial ageing. It's no wonder that mothers with their daughters in the streets of Europe are regularly mistaken for sisters!

Anti-ageing supplements are not just for the face. They treat the whole body to provide us with stronger immunity from disease, enhanced wellbeing and longevity. Supplements can also be used to fix specific problems such as cellulite or weight gain. They treat the face, thighs, buttocks, stomach region and – inside the body – the brain, heart, digestive and immune systems, liver and the like.

Supplements make the face tighter, fuller and with fewer creases. It can also be treated with the essential molecules needed for a natural face-lift effect. Dry and dehydrated skin can be eradicated, and itchy, red, acne-prone skin saved from further outbreaks.

The thighs are a major problem for women. Many get past their teens and no longer feel confident enough to show their legs on the beach in the holiday season. The cause is cellulite. Yet anti-ageing pills can provide the body with components to wipe away that horrid orange-peel skin by turning it into a fat-burning, cellulite-shifting machine. The buttocks are another cause for anxiety because of weight accumulated over the years. Supplements can help to fix that, too.

Weight gain is of paramount concern not just to people on a quest to beat ageing. You can, however, trick the body into a false sense that the stomach is full by stopping the desire to eat through suppressing appetite and take in supplements to help boost metabolism, burn fat and lose pounds.

Organs inside the body age over decades: we suffer a loss of bone minerals, muscle tissue, joint mobility, sexual function, as well as declining immunity to disease, loss of memory and brain function. You can defy almost every part of this degeneration with supplements by incorporating the Dr Nirdosh Anti-Ageing Supplements Plan into your daily schedule. This chapter will reveal what you need to help restore your face back to youth and enjoy a greater sex drive. Now discover how you too can join the exclusive European club of ageless beauties.

The plan requires daily anti-ageing supplements to treat your face and body to a needle-free lift effect. You will discover which work on the face, helping it to fight ageing, and which are vital for the body. Treating internal damage in this way can transform how you look, from head to toe.

The cocktail of youth pills feed the skin with nutrients that encourage internal tightening and lifting. You may have dabbled in them before after hearing of their anti-ageing benefits, but that's not good enough: you must use the right combination at the same time so they work on different parts of the face and body.

High-quality nutrients have been engineered to go deep into the skin layers and aid recovery. Regular use of the supplements will show vast improvements in the skin and body. Cumulative use of unique supplements will help give you back your youthful looks. Now let's look at these wonder pills in detail.

Collagen

Collagen-replenishing capsules feed your skin and body with components to make up for losses of this substance, providing an immediate supply of new collagen to help plump up the skin, which becomes thin, fragile and saggy as it loses its tensile strength with age.

Wrinkles advance through loss of anti-ageing hormones, reduced cell turnover, chronic inflammation and collagen fibres, permanently cross-linking because of Advanced Glycation End products (AGEs). Replenishing collagen – the skin's scaffolding – is vital to ensure that taut, unlined and youthful-looking skin is preserved. Since collagen makes up about 85 per cent of the skin, re-boosting supplies with external anti-ageing collagen supplements is vital. That support can help turn back time damage, plump up wrinkles and give the complexion more resilience.

This is a must-have youth remedy for a natural, needle-free lift. Collagen capsules are widely available, but few have the components to maximise new production. Capsules containing collagen, centella asciatica and vitamin C provide an effective combination of the nutrients needed to help enhance collagen levels. Prolonged use helps to mimic the effects of collagen injections, but without a needle.

Vitamin C (RDA 60mg)

Vitamin C helps healing and has a great effect on the face. Associated with fighting colds and flu, it also aids rapid repair – exactly what we need for the face and body.

Vitamin C helps boost many of our tissues and cells, especially collagen, so accelerating the healing of wounds and defying wrinkle formation. It works by increasing synthesis of the connective tissue collagen. In fact, without vitamin C, collagen formation cannot effectively take place.

Since collagen – found in bone and skin – is the most abundant protein in the body, we need to take it in a supplement. Without it, the collagen capsules will have little impact.

Vitamin C increases longevity and helps fight oxidative damage. To illustrate this first hand, take two bowls of fruit salad. Pour orange juice over the fruit in one of the bowls to completely cover the contents and leave the other as it is. Put both bowls in the fridge. Go back a few days later and you will see that the one without orange juice has started to rot, but the fruit soaked in the juice is probably still as good. That's because the juice-covered fruit has neutralised the free radicals that cause oxidation and ageing.

This power of vitamin C as an antioxidant can counteract age damage so the fruit salad lives on. Similarly, the inner body organs and skin can be protected with it. We will use this supplement to help achieve a firmer, more radiant complexion, a stronger immune system and better all-round health.

Antioxidant Age Block

The effect of antioxidants is powerful too and must be used in a supplement plan to help the face-lift effect. They protect the skin from damage as it is pounded daily by ageing, pollution, our food and the rays of the sun.

These enemies of the skin cause a tiny electron reaction in our cells and make them seemingly go crazy. Some recover, while some are left unstable, injured and incomplete. What we have just experienced is free-radical damage, and the more of it that we experience, the quicker we age. We must block this process with effective antioxidants. They neutralise this reaction and help counteract the free-radical damage. Taking a high-strength antioxidant complex with vitamin A in the form of beta-carotene, vitamins C and E, OPCs and resveratrol is a powerful blend that helps protect skin cells and the internal body from free-radical attack, keeping everything in a healthier, younger state.

Resveratrol also helps preserve healthy collagen and elasticity levels, and it may even be able to switch on SIRT 1, the longevity gene. A specialised complex like this can help give you a younger complexion and body, and even increase your longevity.

You must find an antioxidant complex geared to block ageing

– a powerful anti-ageing supplement that contains an array of specific antioxidants in one capsule will act as a true age block.

Vitamin A (RDA for men: 0.7mg; for women 0.6mg)

Vitamin A is crucial for the skin and body. Foods such as broccoli and carrots contain this vitamin, which encourages good health, longevity and beauty; it is also a potent wrinkle-fighter. Normally, vegetables that are orange or green in colour contain carotene and that's the special molecular component that turns into vitamin A when eaten. It could be debated that food sources should be a first option, but vitamin A is known to be such an effective anti-ageing supplement that, if you don't consume the Recommended Daily Allowance (RDA) of vitamin A from vegetables, then you need to ensure that you get this from a supplement as the benefits can be hugely rewarding.

Initially known as a vitamin good for healthy eye care and vision, this supplement is fantastic at healing wrinkles. It works directly on the epithelial tissue (the openings of passageways to our skin and body). Having the correct amount also allows the body to use it as a powerful antioxidant that helps resist ageing and prevents facial decay; it also assists in collagen preservation and the treatment of acne. After the age of 50, when nutrient absorption can become defective, adding vitamin A as a nutritional supplement is key as it maintains the health of the mucosal membranes, including those in the mouth, digestive system and lungs.

In the body, vitamin A preserves and protects cell membranes; it also helps good liver functionality and protects against heart disease, but the most noticeable effects are in the eye region. Vitamin A is needed for visual adjustment allowing the body to differentiate between light and dark; it also helps prevent the formation of cataracts and encourages good, clear vision to be retained. It's essential to take the correct amount of vitamin A – too much can have a negative effect. The RDA must not be exceeded or the body can suffer toxicity, resulting in headaches, dry skin and blurred vision.

Vitamin E (RDA 10mg)

Many of you will have heard of vitamin E, but may wonder why it is essential to our plan. The vitamin is a fat-soluble antioxidant and, therefore, a key player. Loss of vitamin E is normally associated with the onset of lines and wrinkles. A regular intake of it will show on the face as it can help to smooth lines, wrinkles, scars, stretch marks, sun damage, dry skin and solar lentigines.

Be sure to buy a vitamin E supplement containing D-alpha-tocopherol, as this is the most biologically natural, useable form.

Oestrogen Replacement

Oestrogen is a female hormone progressively lost with age, especially after the menopause. This may cause sagging skin and wrinkles. Soya complexes can mimic the effects of oestrogen because the isoflavones they contain provide cells with phytoestrogens. These can latch on to oestrogen receptors on cells and are therefore seen as a natural form of Hormone Replacement Therapy (HRT).

Oestrogen replacement can help to improve dry, thinning and

creased, drooping skin and female loss of libido, which is why the soya complexes must be integrated into the face-lift programme, especially if you are over 50.

Omega 3, 6 and 9

Skin is highly dependent on lipids – oils – and moisture levels. If these decline, an array of problems surface, from dehydration to dryness and cracking. They may not seem like a big deal, but youthful skin fights hard to keep its natural oils as this delays wrinkle formation. Dry, dehydrated skin becomes lined and ages quickly. This must be defeated with an EFA complex containing omega 3, 6 and 9 to replenish lipid levels.

The rise of natural-oils levels will help soften lines and wrinkles, while alleviating skin-inflammation conditions such as dermatitis, eczema and psoriasis. This vital anti-ageing supplement does its job well and keeps the skin supple, smoother and fuller. EFAs are also essential to combat ageing within the body. Omega 3 and 6 are EFAs that cannot be generated by the body so must be supplied through diet or supplementation. They help maintain joint mobility and brain function, reduce internal inflammation, enhance mood and boost fat loss.

Alpha Lipoic Acid plus Acetyl L Carnitine

The special anti-ageing ingredient, alpha lipoic acid, works effectively in water and fat. This allows it to protect the exterior and interior of a cell by providing a barrier for the fatty skin-cell membrane as well as the interior aqueous environment of the cell. None of the other antioxidants gives this double protection.

So, when you're out and about, this superpower provides your face with nutrients to help you look younger. This encourages prolonged cell life, slows wrinkle formation and helps maintain elasticity and firmness. It can also enhance the function of a substance called glutathione, an antioxidant produced by the body to help it eliminate harmful material, including free radicals. In brain tissue, it helps prevent memory impairment, while in the body it enhances effectiveness of other antioxidants such as vitamins E and C, which are needed for effective collagen production.

Superior supplementation is one containing the powers of alpha lipoic acid and acetyl L carnitine in one capsule, as this combination can actually help lift the face and body. Acetyl L carnitine acts by boosting levels of the neuro-transmitter acetylcholine. This can stimulate the facial muscles to contract, making them lift and appear firmer. It can also contract the body muscles, such as those of the buttocks and thighs, giving both bum and body a tighter, lifted look. This is amazing – this supplement is now working to help your face- and body-lift! In time, it can help tighten the facial muscles to provide a natural, needle-free face- and body-lift effect, directly combating facial and body sagging.

If you want a potent anti-ageing mix that can help enhance a face-lift effect, you need alpha lipoic acid and acetyl L carnitine combined together.

Youth-Restoring Growth Hormone Booster

If I were to give you a potion to thicken your skin, eradicate lines, repair age damage, enhance fat loss and boost muscle tissue, would you want it? Welcome to Human Growth Hormone in a capsule! Hailed by celebrities and journalists as the miracle youth pill, it turns back the clock to make the body look younger.

We all have Human Growth Hormone in our bodies, but its levels deplete with age and we start to degenerate. This miracle anti-ageing supplement can give you an instant Growth Hormone boost as it contains the desired amino acid complex to help rebuild this hormone. By doing this, your body can remain in an anti-ageing state. The results of the Growth Hormone-boosting supplements can make you look miraculously young and beautiful. Capsules are not widely available and most people do not even know that such a powerful supplement exists.

It is regularly taken by high-profile sports personalities and celebrities. They know their bodies are always on the go and vulnerable to damage that accelerates ageing. Taking external doses of Growth Hormone-enhancing complexes keeps their bodies young. It feeds their face and body cells with Growth Hormone boosters so they don't suffer the signs of ageing.

This is probably the most important anti-ageing supplement on the plan. Added to my cocktail of anti-ageing remedies, you have the complete prescription of supplements to inject youth and beauty back into your face and body.

COMPLETE VITAMIN B COMPLEX

Complete vitamin B complex is a special universal anti-ageing supplement. It is labelled a complex because it comprises eight individual vitamin B components, each of them unique and specific to its task.

B vitamins are needed to maintain a healthy nervous system, metabolism, energy production, red blood cells, healthy skin and muscle tissue. A lack of them is apparent as sores and cracks appear around the mouth, the mood is lowered and you become irritable, with lapses of memory, lethargy, acne, skin rashes and itchiness plus thinning hair. The body cannot create all the B vitamins itself so it has to get them from external sources which is why this is more than an anti-ageing pill.

Let's look at what the components do and remember that all the benefits and the eight different parts of the complete vitamin B complex are crammed into one tablet.

Vitamin B1 (RDA for men 1mg; for women 0.8mg)

Known as thiamine, its importance lies in converting carbohydrates to energy, as well as promoting nerve, heart and muscle health. Thiamine's function in combating ageing is crucial as it prevents breakdown of the central nervous system as well as protecting the skin from lesions and maintaining muscle tone.

Vitamin B2 – Riboflavin (RDA for men 1.3mg; for women 1.1mg)

This is responsible for the health of the skin, nails, hair, nervous and immune systems, as well as cell metabolism. It helps to keep the eye lenses in good condition and can help prevent cataracts, a common eye problem linked to ageing. On a smaller scale, too little riboflavin can cause conjunctivitis.

Like most of the other B vitamins, its primary function is

energy production from food. Riboflavin helps increase the potency of other antioxidants like vitamin E and glutathione, so it increases cell protection against oxidation damage.

Vitamin B3 – Niacin (RDA for men 17mg; for women 13mg)

Niacin is especially important in regulating some digestive functions as it plays a role in insulin stabilisation. It has been shown to lower levels of LDL by decreasing their release from adipose (fat) tissue, so it helps lowers bad cholesterol.

Vitamin B5 – Pantothenic Acid (RDA 6mg)

Especially important for its ability to calm acne and control sebum production, when vitamin B5 is present, skin wounds can heal better and the pores have a better chance of normalising. B5 also helps strengthen hair and provides energy by optimising the digestion of food.

Vitamin B6 – Pyridoxine (RDA for men 1.4mg; for women 1.2mg)

Vitamin B6 is a co-factor, which speeds up hundreds of inner-body reactions. Especially important in brain neurotransmitter activity, it is involved in the production of serotonin, melatonin and dopamine.

In women, it helps alleviate pre-menstrual tension and symptoms of breast tenderness, fluid retention, moodiness and skin breakouts by stabilising hormone levels and prostaglandins. As an anti-ageing molecule, B6 helps repel the production of homocysteine, a chemical that damages the cardiovascular system and lining of blood vessels.

Vitamin B7 – Biotin (RDA 0.15mg)

This important B vitamin regulates cell growth and keeps skin and hair healthy. It is really important for skin-cell health as a deficiency can lead to defective cell walls, which results in inflammatory disorders and accelerates ageing.

Vitamin B9 – Folic Acid (RDA 0.2mg)

Folic acid is a vital molecule heavily involved in cellular growth and division. It helps keep blood healthy as it is needed in the process of erythropoiesis – formation of red blood cells, as well as production of white blood cells. It is also especially important for a developing foetus. In fact, the British government recommends pregnant women take 0.4mg a day of folic acid for 12 weeks prior to conception.

Too little increases the risk of neural tube defects such as spina bifida and other congenital defects like cleft palate. Folic acid may have a role in promoting division and growth of fibroblasts, cells in the skin's dermis that make collagen and elastin.

Vitamin B9's ability to regenerate fibroblasts and reduce DNA damage makes it a powerful defence against ageing. It can also help skin cells heal from UV damage and enhance photo-protection.

Vitamin B12 – Cyanocoalbumin (RDA 0.0015mg)

This affects nearly every cell in our bodies and is critically involved in preserving our DNA. Its role in healthy cell division is vital: it helps preserve the myelin sheath that covers nerve cells and affects certain neurotransmitters in the brain. Loss of this can increase depression and neuronal damage, reduce our energy, make us gain weight and accelerates stress. This readily accessible vitamin is often overlooked, but it must go into your anti-ageing supplement prescription.

Zinc Gluconate (RDA 15mg)

Zinc is a healer, aiding recovery from within. Most importantly, it helps regenerate healthy DNA, boosts immunity and wound repairs so your body will benefit from a supplement that helps it to simultaneously mend damaged cells of the face and body, while boosting immune defences to give you robust health.

The molecular components of zinc speed up the wound-curing process and that includes facial skin. It is needed for regeneration of collagen, so this is a must if you want to help your face and body maintain firmness. Zinc also effectively helps to control excess sebum production and treats skin conditions that affect the appearance of the face such as acne, eczema and psoriasis. It will help correct enlarged skin pores, which occur in teens and in maturing skin.

Co-enzyme Q10

Lab tests show this amazing supplement can boost the immune system and lengthen our youth and lifespan. Levels decline with age and, as they do so, so too does our overall health. Its benefits are widely accepted in countries such as Japan – the Japanese know that taking it as a daily anti-ageing supplement can help the body back to youth.

Q10 is associated with energy, and the more energy the body requires, the more Q10 it needs. This is because Q10 is present in nearly every cell and it enhances the metabolic processes. The ability to enhance new cell turnover makes it critical for ageing skin, as it can counteract declining production and define a renewed complexion.

It also helps promote a healthy metabolism and weight loss. Having ample Q10 in your body ensures a healthy heart and lung function, as these require energy to work. Taking this supplement daily can have astonishing benefits and is a requirement of my anti-ageing plan.

Pomegranate with Ellagic Acid

One good pomegranate tablet containing ellagic acid can provide the equivalent of eight glasses of pomegranate juice. This is a magical free-radical fighter that works on both the face and body. It also provides wider health benefits, such as anti-mutagenic and anti-cancerous support to help protect the genetic material in skin cells from disease and promote a longer, healthier life. Ellagic acid also helps shield against UV rays, providing vital anti-ageing support to the skin in assisting to enhance defensive barriers.

Goji Berry

The highest on the ORAC Scale – which measures oxygen radical absorptive capacity – goji is a true leader in the fight against ageing. It may even contain Growth Hormone Secretagogues that signal to the body to secrete the youth hormone and can help stop wrinkles from forming. Those living in the Himalayas have taken goji for generations and have record levels of life expectancy.

Weight Loss and Cellulite

The reason we have a weight-loss pill is that age slows down metabolism and fat-burning mechanisms, which results in weight gain and cellulite for women. We must keep active as we age, as this allows the body to beat conditions such as obesity. The correct anti-ageing pill can help you lose weight and combat cellulite.

The trick is to use special supplements that include green tea, caffeine and chromium, a combination that will ignite thermogenesis – a process that fuels internal fat burning. Areas like the abdomen, thighs, buttocks and cellulite can be treated in this way. This will help the body shed adipose tissue, as the formulation of the fat-burning pill helps break down fat from problematic areas. The combination is essential to create a lean, youthful body.

For weight loss you also need a supplement that can help suppress the appetite and creates a false sense of fullness. Ingredients such as hoodia (see page 176) settle unnecessary bingeing and help reduce overall calorie intake without your feeling hunger pangs. This kind of action makes dieting a breeze. So, for dramatic leanness, as well as taking an appetite suppressant, combine this with a supplement with the ingredients described above to give weight and fat loss a mega-boost.

Hoodia

This anti-ageing supplement is crucial in our quest to make the body younger. It works to beat the fight against weight gain and fat accumulation. Hoodia cleverly tricks the body into thinking that it is full through its appetite-suppressant properties. The P57 molecule it contains is an active component that works to alter ATP, an energy molecule in the body that can affect hunger pangs. Adding this supplement to the plan means that you will not only start to look younger, but you'll also begin to rapidly lose weight.

Hoodia works in two ways: first, it allows your body to promote lipolysis (fat loss) and it also minimises food cravings. Hoodia promotes thermogenic action, a fat-burning process inside the body, which will allow you to drop a dress size fast. This doubly powerful combination is the perfect process when you want your body to become leaner and to rid yourself of excess weight. By stopping food cravings and turning the body into a fat-burning machine, you instantly become healthier and far more agile as you eradicate excess calories. On our quest to de-age the body and face and to create a svelte figure, this is the perfect anti-ageing supplement to make it possible.

Calcium and Vitamin D

Renowned for helping to keep bones and teeth strong, calcium's role in beautifying the skin isn't quite so well known. In fact, it enhances a more resilient, firmer complexion and promotes skin regeneration by encouraging cell division, so protecting against the formation of age lines, thinning skin and wrinkle development. It helps to smooth the outermost keratin layer of the skin by enhancing cell turnover and also forms part of fibroblasts responsible for collagen production, so it helps enhance collagen renewal and plays a role in retaining tensile strength of skin. This is vital as the skin ages because not only do we lose existing collagen but also production becomes defective due to a lack of certain substances such as calcium. As we age, calcium is crucial to keep the facial skin supported and it is also a vital requirement for sturdy, healthy nails, strong teeth and bone mineralisation as it protects against osteoporosis.

Without vitamin D, the body cannot effectively absorb calcium, so it will suffer deficiency. That's why it's essential to include vitamin D in the plan.

Lycopene

Lycopene is a carotenoid antioxidant that gives food its rich orange-red colour. Naturally, it is rich in tomatoes. As the body cannot manufacture it, it must be consumed from external sources to gain the benefits of this powerful antioxidant and receive the right amount daily. The power of lycopene lies in its ability to combat free radicals and shield against UV ageing radiation, especially from the sun. This action helps keep the skin firm and youthful.

Lycopene also helps the body retain good health and works hard to protect against major diseases, such as cancer of the prostate, lungs and digestive system. A specialist longevity enhancer, it can shield against face and body ageing.

Green Tea

If you ever want a quick and effective anti-ageing boost, look no further than green tea. This super anti-ageing supplement can be hailed nothing short of a miracle for its long list of effective anti-ageing benefits. The reason why it's so good is because it's rich in Epigallocatechin Gallates (EGCGs). These highly powerful antioxidants are known to be more potent than vitamins C and E, and will bolster the immune system as well as improve overall skin health. The anti-inflammatory action of the catechins in green tea help fend off viruses, eliminate free-radical molecules, prevent cellular deterioration and protect against UV radiation by yielding a sunscreen barrier effect, which means that the green tea EGCGs can work to slow down the formation of wrinkles and protect the body from serious medical illnesses.

The reason why green tea is included as a supplement rather than a drink is because the supplement can eliminate the caffeine part of green tea, which means you get all the advantages of green tea minus the stimulant effect. Green tea also has a de-stressing effect. It is an integral part of the anti-ageing supplement plan.

So, the combined effort of the above supplements works on specific parts of the face and body, targeting the core of the problem from the inside out. Some supplements work on wrinkles, others tackle collagen levels, plumping skin or helping to thicken skin or fight sagging, while one even helps to lift the face itself. For the body, some supplements boost immunity,

The Dr Nirdosh Anti-Ageing Supplements Plan

Anti-Ageing Supplement Plan			
THE ANTI-AGEING NEEDLE-FREE FACE-LIFT		**THE ANTI-AGEING NEEDLE-FREE BODY-LIFT**	
Collagen Capsules	Benefit: Enhances collagen	Complete Vitamin B Complex	Benefit: Universal body-repairing vitamin, gives energy, maintains healthy nervous system and skin
Vitamin C	Benefit: Accelerates repair, including wrinkles and collagen, while giving the immune system a mighty boost	Zinc Gluconate	Benefit: Heals wounds and helps regenerate healthy DNA. Useful for skin and body repair
Antioxidant Complex	Benefit: Blocks ageing and slows down further ageing	Co-enzyme Q10	Benefit: Extends life and enhances new cell production
Vitamin E	Benefit: Smoothes wrinkles and lines, diminishes sun damage, skin scars and stretch marks	Pomegranate	Benefit: Blocks age damage in the body and protects DNA
Omega 3, 6 and 9	Benefit: Keeps skin moisture boosted and supple; fights lines, thinning and dry, crackly skin and wrinkles	Goji berry	Benefit: Extends youth and longevity in the whole body
Vitamin A	Benefit: Combats acne, treats hyperpigmentation and wrinkles, enhances cell production, renews the skin's surface and maintains healthy, clear vision	Green tea plus caffeine, plus chromium	Benefit: Assists in rapid weight loss, especially from the buttocks, thighs and abdominal regions

Anti-Ageing Supplement Plan (cont.)			
THE ANTI-AGEING NEEDLE-FREE FACE-LIFT		**THE ANTI-AGEING NEEDLE-FREE BODY-LIFT**	
Alpha Lipoic	Benefit: Slows wrinkle formation, repairs and protects skin cells; preserves brain function. Recycles other antioxidants, including vitamin C, necessary for collagen production	Soya Complex	Benefit: Mimics the effects of oestrogen and fights skin sagging
Acetyl L Carnitine	Benefit: Lifts the face and body; enhances cell turnover	Hoodia	Benefit: Enhances weight loss and tricks the body into a false sense of feeling full
Lycopene	Benefit: Boosts the skin's natural sunscreen, provides potent antioxidant support and resists disease	Growth Hormone Boosters	Benefit: Thickens skin, reduces line formation, promotes fat loss, enhances muscle tissue, strengthens bones, boosts immunity and combats ageing
Green Tea	Benefit: Enhances defences against sun and pollution damage, de-stresses mind, neutralises oxidative damage and promotes weight loss	Calcium and Vitamin D	Benefit: Enhances resilience of bones, nails and teeth; helps to enhance a firmer complexion by promoting collagen renewal

others enhance longevity and get rid of cellulite or help you to burn fat and lose weight. Introducing them into your lifestyle with daily use will help you to achieve a natural body- and face-lift without any need to go near the surgeon's knife.

There is one dilemma that we must now address, something that may until now have stopped you from following an anti-ageing treatment plan for yourself: how many supplements am I meant to use each day and which ones do I take when? Already you have the vital list of special anti-ageing supplements that you need. As we have already discussed, the skin and body work differently at various stages in life and it is therefore unnecessary to include every single anti-ageing supplement in your plan.

However, it's a question that I always come across and the Dr Nirdosh Anti-Ageing Supplements Plan is the first to give you an exact plan for your face and body age. Instead of thinking, how many pills am I meant to pop and which ones are correct for my age, simply look at the chart. As your skin and body change, adjust the plan so you know that you are always using the most effective supplements for your age.

This Anti-Ageing Supplements Plan has been developed to ensure that at any given time your body and face receive the vital substances they need to repair, heal, protect and even reverse internal ageing, as this is normally where the damage occurs. Following the unique plan means that you can just get on with life, knowing that you are taking steps to ensure your body always performs at its optimum levels and fends off ageing.

The Anti-Ageing Supplement Prescription Chart
Age 20–35

Take the following supplements on the Dr Nirdosh Plan if you fall into this age profile. They will extend your body's ability to fight ageing while capitalising on your youth and agility.

Vitamin C aims to…
- Enhance collagen synthesis
- Create a radiant, even complexion by combating rough and bumpy, dull skin
- Neutralise free radicals that damage healthy cells and environmental toxins that cause ageing
- Slow down ageing in the face and body
- Strengthen the immune system better to fight infections and diseases
- Protect against sun damage.

Vitamin B complex aims to…
- Allow optimum metabolism of vital food nutrients
- Fight off skin-damaging conditions such as acne, oily skin and rosacea
- Heal skin complications such as rashes
- Preserve healthy hair
- Boost energy levels and combat irritability and fatigue
- Help organs such as the skin, digestive system, liver and brain to perform
- Boost the nervous system, brain capabilities, memory and alertness.

The Dr Nirdosh Anti-Ageing Supplements Plan

Zinc gluconate aims to...

- Speed up wound and skin healing
- Keep the complexion clear
- Control acne breakouts
- Heal eczema-type skin conditions, including psoriasis
- Help regenerate collagen
- Maintain skin firmness
- Help heal internal body damage.

Age block antioxidant complex with beta-carotene and resveratrol aims to...

- Activate the anti-ageing gene SIRT 1
- Help extend youth and life
- Improve health and beauty
- Block ageing free radicals
- Guard against pollution and sun damage
- Protect the skin and body from ageing attacks
- Resveratrol helps preserve healthy collagen for a firmer, smoother face.

Vitamin E aims to...

- Define a supple complexion
- Help smooth fine lines and wrinkles
- Heal and soften scars and stretch marks
- Protect against sun damage
- Preserve a healthy cardiovascular system
- Improve healthy brain function.

Omega 3 aims to…

- Help anti-inflammatory action in the skin and body
- Boost moisture levels
- Replenish oils
- Soften wrinkles
- Strengthen hair
- Enhance fat burning
- Promote healthy brain function
- Maintain active bone joints
- Improve mood.

Pomegranate with ellagic acid aims to…

- Prevent internal DNA damage
- Protect against sun damage
- Fend off pollution damage
- Offer protection from diseases, including cancer
- Promote longevity
- Encourage healthier skin and body.

Lycopene aims to…

- Provide sun-blocking filter for UVA and UVB broad-spectrum protection
- Guard the face against external ageing
- Provide mega-powerful antioxidant action to help destroy free radicals
- Help protect the body against diseases such as cancer.

Green tea EGCGs aim to...
- Enhance protection against sun and pollution
- Fend off ageing
- Act as defence against cancer
- Enhance a younger, more beautiful complexion
- Elevate metabolism and fat burning
- Combat stress and anxiety
- Induce calm
- Sharpen the mind.

Age 35–50

If you are between 35 and 50, these pills will counteract the ageing that is likely to show on your face and body by now. My specific prescription will refuel and prime your face and body with vital lost nutrients to help slow down the ageing process and turn back some of the signs of damage. The plan aims to allow the face and body to return to youth and beauty. Part of this plan includes some supplements prescribed for skin aged 20–35. However, there are additional ones that target specific concerns for this age category.

Vitamin C aims to...
- Enhance collagen synthesis
- Create a radiant, even complexion while combating rough and bumpy, dull skin
- Neutralise free radicals that damage healthy cells and environmental toxins that cause ageing
- Slow ageing in the face and body

- Strengthen the immune system to better fight infections and diseases
- Protect against sun damage.

Vitamin B Complex aims to…
- Allow optimum metabolism of vital food nutrients
- Fight off damaging skin conditions such as acne, oily skin and rosacea
- Heal skin complications like rashes
- Preserve healthy hair
- Boost energy levels and combat irritability and fatigue
- Help organs such as the skin, digestive system, liver and brain to perform
- Boost the nervous system, brain capabilities, memory and alertness.

Zinc gluconate aims to…
- Speed up healing of wounds
- Maintain a clear complexion
- Control outbreaks of acne
- Heal eczema-type skin conditions, including psoriasis
- Help regenerate collagen, maintain skin firmness and heal internal body damage.

Age block antioxidant complex with beta-carotene and resveratrol aims to…
- Activate the anti-ageing gene SIRT 1
- Help to extend youth and life

- Improve health and beauty
- Block ageing free radicals
- Guard against pollution and sun damage
- Protect the skin and body from ageing attacks
- Resveratrol helps preserve healthy collagen for a firmer, smoother face.

Powerful EFA supplement is a complex of omega 3, 6 and 9, plus vitamin E preferably in one capsule. The aims of the separate components are listed below.

Omega 3 aims to...
- Perform an anti-inflammatory action in the skin and body
- Boost moisture levels
- Replenish oil levels
- Diminish wrinkles
- Strengthen and maintain glossy hair
- Enhance fat burning
- Promote healthy brain function
- Maintain active bone joints and a healthy cardiovascular system
- Improve mood.

Omega 6 aims to...
- Maintain regular hormonal balance
- Combat pre-menstrual tension
- Keep the heart healthy
- Aid memory
- Revive dull, dry skin

- Smooth fine lines and keep skin supple, alleviating inflammation
- Tackle dermatitis, eczema and psoriasis
- Maintain strong and shiny hair.

Omega 9 aims to...
- Keep skin young and healthy
- Nourish hair and keep it strong
- Ensure a healthy brain and heart.

Vitamin E aims to...
- Help define a supple complexion
- Help smooth fine lines and wrinkles
- Heal and soften scars and stretch marks
- Protect against sun damage
- Preserve a healthy cardiovascular system
- Improve brain health.

Co-enzyme Q10 aims to...
- Prolong youth and life by boosting the production of new cells
- Speed up cell metabolism
- Improve energy levels
- Encourage weight loss
- The antioxidant action fights ageing molecules.

Alpha Lipoic Acid + Acetyl L Carnitine complex
The alpha lipoic acid components of this complex aim to...

- Block ageing by protecting the inner and outer parts of cells
- Prolong youth by helping to extend healthy cell life
- Help halt wrinkle formation
- Tighten and firm up the face
- Recycle antioxidants, turning the body into an age-defending machine
- Prevent memory impairment
- Help reproduce skin collagen by enhancing vitamin C activity.

The acetyl L carnitine components aim to…
- Give a natural face-lift
- Tighten body muscles
- Combat skin sagging
- Make skin more youthful
- Improve concentration
- Boost metabolism and weight loss
- Shift cellulite
- Smooth and lift the bum.

Collagen capsules
The components of this complex aim to…
- Plump and tighten the face
- Fill wrinkles
- Lift sagging skin
- Decrease scar tissue
- Promote wound repair
- Strengthen nails and hair

- Resist skin thinning.

Growth Hormone boosting complex
The components of this complex aim to…
- Make the body look younger with an anti-ageing hormone enhancer
- Inject youth back into the body by replenishing lost Growth Hormone
- Improve skin thickness
- Reduce wrinkles
- Tighten and firm the face
- Increase muscle tissue and tone
- Produce a trimmer, tighter body
- Strengthen bones
- Promote fat and weight loss
- Halt ageing in the whole face and body.

Goji berries aim to…
- Prolong youth and enhance longevity
- Help block ageing (on the ORAC Scale, it's the leader as the most powerful antioxidant)
- Protect the skin and body from ageing.

Pomegranate with ellagic acid aims to…
- Prevent internal DNA damage
- Protect against sun damage
- Fend off pollution damage
- Protect against cancer and other diseases

- Promote longevity
- Encourage healthier skin and body.

Lycopene aims to...

- Provide sun-blocking filter for UVA and UVB broad-spectrum rays
- Guard the face against external ageing
- Destroy free radicals
- Help protect against diseases, among them cancer.

Green tea EGCGs aim to...

- Enhance protection against UV rays, sun and pollution damage
- Fend off ageing
- Provide anti-carcinogenic activity
- Enhance a younger, more beautiful complexion
- Elevate metabolism and fat burning
- Combat stress and anxiety
- Induce calm.

Cellulite supplement with green tea, caffeine and chromium (preferably one capsule as a powerful anti-cellulite and weight loss complex)

The components aim to...

- Turn the body into a fat-burning machine
- Boost metabolism and fat loss (lipolysis)
- Prevent food cravings and binges
- Stabilise blood-sugar levels.

Age 50

Skin in its fifties has reached a turning point that requires extra care and attention. More than ever, the anti-ageing supplements must be an essential part of your plan and lifestyle. The body relies on them as the internal mechanism for manufacturing vital vitamins, nutrients, minerals and hormones at youthful levels has evaporated. This leaves a dangerous void, exposing the body to harsh environmental factors that precipitate ageing. To avoid accelerated ageing and age-related diseases, implement anti-ageing supplements for six weeks as this will not only fight ageing concerns, but also provide lost micronutrients that the body relies on to function well.

The anti-ageing supplements will work to give you back your youth, vitality and health, behind a maturing body and face.

Vitamin C aims to…
- Enhance collagen synthesis
- Create a radiant, even complexion while combating rough and bumpy, dull skin
- Neutralise free radicals that damage healthy cells and environmental toxins that cause ageing
- Slow ageing in the body and face
- Strengthen the immune system to better fight infections and diseases
- Protect against sun damage.

Vitamin B complex aims to…
- Allow optimum metabolism of vital food nutrients

- Fight off skin-damaging conditions such as acne, oily skin and rosacea
- Heal skin complications such as rashes
- Preserve healthy hair
- Boost energy levels and combat irritability and fatigue
- Assist organs such as the skin, digestive system, liver and brain to perform optimally
- Boost the nervous system, brain capabilities, memory and alertness.

Zinc gluconate aims to…
- Speed up wound and skin healing
- Maintain a clear complexion
- Control acne breakouts
- Heal eczema-type conditions including psoriasis
- Help regenerate collagen and maintain skin firmness
- Help heal internal body damage.

Age block antioxidant complex with beta-carotene and resveratrol aims to…
- Activate the anti-ageing gene SIRT 1
- Help extend youth and life
- Improve health and beauty
- Block ageing free radicals
- Guard against pollution and sun damage
- Protect the skin and body from ageing attacks
- Resveratrol helps preserve healthy collagen for a firmer, smoother face.

Powerful EFA supplement: complex of omega 3, 6 and 9, plus vitamin E, preferably all in one capsule. The aims of the components are listed below.

Omega 3 aims to…

- Produce an anti-inflammatory action in the skin and body
- Boost moisture levels
- Replenish oil levels
- Diminish wrinkles
- Strengthen and maintain glossy hair
- Enhance fat burning
- Promote healthy brain function
- Maintain active bone joints and a healthy cardiovascular system
- Improve mood.

Omega 6 aims to…

- Maintain regular hormonal balance
- Combat pre-menstrual tension
- Keep the heart healthy
- Aid memory
- Revive dull, dry skin
- Smooth fine lines and keep skin supple, alleviating inflammation
- Tackle dermatitis, eczema and psoriasis
- Maintain strong and shiny hair.

Omega 9 aims to…

- Keep skin young and healthy

- Nourish hair and keep it strong
- Ensure a healthy brain and heart.

Vitamin E aims to…
- Help define a supple complexion
- Help smooth fine lines and wrinkles
- Heal and soften scars and stretch marks
- Protect against sun damage
- Preserve a healthy cardiovascular system
- Improve brain health.

Alpha lipoic acid and acetyl L carnitine combined complex
The alpha lipoic components aim to…
- Block ageing by protecting inner and outer cells
- Prolong youth by helping to extend healthy cell life
- Help halt wrinkle formation
- Tighten and firm the face
- Recycle antioxidants, reusing them to turn the body into an age-defending machine
- Prevent memory impairment
- Help reproduce skin collagen by enhancing vitamin C activity.

The acetyl L carnitine components aim to…
- Give a natural face-lift
- Tighten body muscles
- Combat sagging skin and make it look more youthful
- Improve concentration
- Boost metabolism and weight loss

- Shift cellulite
- Smooth and lift the bum.

Collagen capsules

The components of this complex aim to…

- Plump and tighten the face
- Fill wrinkles and lift sagging skin
- Decrease scar tissue
- Promote wound repair
- Strengthen nails and hair
- Resist skin thinning.

Growth Hormone-boosting complex

Its components aim to…

- Make the body younger with anti-ageing hormone enhancer
- Inject youth back into the body by replenishing lost Growth Hormone
- Improve skin thickness
- Reduce wrinkles
- Tighten and firm facial skin
- Increase muscle tissue and tone
- Gain a trimmer, tighter body
- Strengthen bones
- Promote fat and weight loss
- Halt ageing in the whole face and body.

Soya complex

Its components aim to…

- Mimic the female hormone oestrogen
- Relieve menopausal losses such as hot flushes
- Strengthen bones
- Put youth back into the body
- Promote fat loss and a reversal of ageing
- Strengthen, smooth and plump up skin
- Combat sagging and rough, dry skin
- Boost libido.

Calcium and vitamin D
The components aim to...
- Enhance collagen renewal for a firmer, better-supported face
- Build agility in the bones and joints
- Make teeth healthy, hair stronger and nails more resilient.

Goji berry
This complex aims to...
- Prolong youth and enhance longevity
- Help block ageing – it's a leader on ORAC Scale, being the most powerful antioxidant
- Protect both skin and body from ageing.

Cellulite supplement with green tea, caffeine and chromium, preferably in one capsule with all the above as a power anti-cellulite, weight-loss complex
The components aim to...
- Transform the body into a fat-burning machine
- Boost metabolism and fat loss (lipolysis)

- Prevent food cravings and binges
- Stabilise blood-sugar levels.

Hoodia appetite suppressant aims to…
- Trick the stomach into thinking that it's full
- Decrease appetite and calorie intake
- Promote weight loss.

Vitamin A aims to…
- Protect skin-cell membranes
- Heal wrinkles and lines
- Rectify acne and other blemishes
- Enhance new cell turnover and a refined complexion
- Treat psoriasis, eczema and dry skin
- Diminish age spots (hyperpigmentation)
- Help combat hair loss and thinning
- Help preserve collagen
- Provide antioxidant support in the body
- Maintain healthy eyes and clear vision
- Prevent skin thinning.

As I mentioned earlier, the aim of taking anti-ageing pills is to make both the face and body look younger and provide the internal mechanisms of the body with the nutrients, vitamins, minerals, antioxidants and hormones it needs to help combat age damage.

Chapter 9
Sleeping Beauty

SLEEP IS JUST as important as any of the other disciplines in this book. The goal on this anti-ageing plan is to make your body refuel itself with youth and beauty, rather than wrinkles and ageing. But sleep is one of the most overlooked parts of anti-ageing and the consequence of not getting your sleep patterns right will leave you lagging behind, with continual age damage, and wondering why the results are not forthcoming because lack of sleep causes internal and visual age damage.

Sleep is paramount to the whole regeneration cycle that the body is involved in during any given 24-hour period and to disrupt this cycle routinely will result in the natural anti-ageing powers of the body diminishing rapidly. It's a process meticulously controlled by a tiny section of the brain known as the pineal gland, which secretes a hormone called melatonin that causes us to feel tranquilised and forces us to rest. Our pattern of sleep and waking is set by the body's 24-hour timer, which allows us to follow a diurnal lifestyle triggered by changes of light and dark so we spend half our day awake and the night-time hours resting.

The amazing thing is that, with the right amount of sleep at the right time, you can actually encourage powerful anti-ageing hormones to be released back into the body while you sleep. This is a practice that high-performance athletes engage in daily because they know the anti-ageing benefits of sleep: they use the power of sleep to help their bodies become younger and stronger. It is common for some sports professionals such as bodybuilders to sleep one to two hours before engaging in their weight-training routines as this power nap forces their bodies to secrete a strength boost, both physically and mentally. Sleep has an anabolic anti-ageing effect as it causes youthful chemicals such as Growth Hormone and melatonin to flood our systems, allowing the body to rebuild and mend itself.

Scientific research has shown that regular sleepers live longer and sleep helps improve the immune system. Sleep deprivation causes ageing due to an imbalanced, ill-repaired body. You feel exhausted, can't think straight, feel groggy, under-perform and increase your chances of heart disease. Skin cells don't recover properly, so wounds and scarring, including wrinkles, line the face and the complexion looks grey, dry and aged. A real sleeping beauty needs to ensure six to eight hours of undisturbed sleep each night!

THE TWO KINDS OF SLEEP

The body sleeps in two ways, which have different effects. These are called NON-REM (non-rapid eye movement) and REM (rapid eye movement) sleep. The combination of NON-REM and REM completes one cycle of sleep which lasts anywhere between 90 and 120 minutes. Throughout the night, we experience about five of these cycles, which forces our body into repair mode when it works to fix daytime wear and tear. Mentally and physically, this process refreshes us so we can tackle the day ahead. Sleep is Nature's free anti-ageing gift and that's why you cannot miss it. Now let's take a look at the two independent ways in which we sleep.

Non-Rapid Eye Movement Sleep (NON-REM)

This is the first type of sleep that we experience and during this phase the brain relaxes and becomes quiet and inactive. Eventually, the muscles relax, breathing slows and the body calms down. There is slight movement, but you will not be aware of this. NON-REM sleep is divided into a further four phases, which we will shortly discuss.

Rapid Eye Movement (REM)

This occurs about 70 to 90 minutes after NON-REM sleep and it's the time when we dream. The reason why it's called Rapid Eye Movement is because during this phase of sleep your brain is quite active, but the body is in a near-paralysed state with the muscles totally relaxed and the eyes moving from side to side. Your body goes through REM sleep about four to five times during the night.

NATURE'S ANTI-AGEING GIFT

The number-one wonder anti-ageing hormone, hailed as 'cosmetic surgery in a capsule', is Growth Hormone. This is the ultimate special age-reversing hormone. Not only does it work hard to reinject youth into the body, but it also fights off the damaging stress hormone cortisol.

A-list celebrities pay over the odds to get Growth Hormone back into their bodies from external sources to ensure levels remain optimised, as the result of Human Growth Hormone can be astounding and includes thicker facial skin, increased muscle mass, increased collagen production, stronger bones, a younger body and a wrinkle-free face. You can get some Growth Hormone naturally starting tonight, provided you get a good night's sleep!

Sleeping properly is vital on the Dr Nirdosh Plan as it reintroduces the anti-ageing hormones Growth Hormone and melatonin into the body. During sleep, the most intense bursts of Growth Hormone release occur. Skip sleep and you miss out on peak anti-ageing hormone activity. The sleep phases have different chemical reactions in our bodies, the most important being Deep Slow Wave NON-REM Sleep Phases 3 and 4. During these hours, the body naturally releases masses of Human Growth Hormone (HGH) via the pituitary gland in the brain. This helps the body to recover, repair and anti-age.

The two parts of sleep (NON-REM and REM) are complicated processes and we now need to look at the split stages in more detail. Let's look at how what happens.

The Four Phases of NON-REM Sleep

During sleep, your brain gradually loses activation and there is strong brain and body connection. It's essential that you do not place your body in a high state of anxiety before bedtime and instead prepare to enter a calm, relaxed state at least an hour before you retire for the day.

Phase One

During this phase, the body and brain go through some dramatic changes as you prepare to engage in sleep. The brain places you in a light sleep, which you slowly drift in and out of. To help induce sleepiness, the body releases the hormone melatonin. The thing to note here is that your body temperature drops, the muscles relax, breathing slows down and your heart rate slows down. At this point the brain also slows down and brain waves change from active alpha waves to calmer theta waves. You become drowsy and may experience twitches. It is important to decelerate about an hour before bedtime as this helps the body regress into the theta wave phase with ease, taking you into a sleep mode. Here, the cycle can easily be interrupted and you may be woken quite readily.

Phase Two

The body falls deeper into sleep and brain activity slows down further. This is a process that lasts about 15–20 minutes when organs such as the heart and lungs experience a real slowdown and body is in a subconscious state. This takes up a lot of sleep time.

Phase Three

Now the body and brain connection change again and this time the body goes into a phase called the delta wave stage, as the brain relaxes even further. This is called Slow Wave Sleep and it is during this stage that it becomes difficult to wake a sleeping person as they have already fallen into a really deep sleep.

Phase Four

This is a continuation of Phase Three in which the brain falls deeper into Slow Wave Sleep and activity is at its most calm.

Phases Three and Four (Slow Wave Sleep) are a golden state as it is in these precious short moments that masses of anti-ageing Human Growth Hormone are released into the body. Sleep floods the body with this youth-fixing hormone so that it has the chemicals to repair and rebuild itself from within – it's here that you are at the core of fighting ageing! Having this beautiful hormone flowing around your body helps you retain vital muscle mass tissue, fight off bone decay, have a good set of healthy, active organs and beat facial wrinkles. It also allows you to enjoy thicker and plumper skin as collagen levels are replenished and healthy skin-cell regeneration can take place. This allows injured or dead skin cells to be replaced with newer or reformed ones. In a nutshell, it stops you ageing and gives your body youth.

If you're not sleeping well or regularly have erratic restlessness due to late nights, the chances are that you are missing your vital Human Growth Hormone release. Stress and our modern lifestyles regularly keep us up at night and now you can see how this causes rapid ageing. If you don't sleep properly, you never experience the full length of Delta Slow wave phase of sleep, so you miss essential recovery every night and instead fast-forward ageing.

REM Sleep

REM occurs right after Phase Four and it's here that you start to dream. Your body enters Rapid Eye Movement sleep and you will start to breathe irregularly. Even your muscles can become temporarily paralysed – 'sleep paralysis'. This phase cuts in about an hour to 90 minutes after falling asleep and lasts for about 10–25 minutes. During REM sleep, brain activity suddenly becomes alert and heart rate and blood pressure change. It's during this phase that both these factors can go up very high, which is why many heart attacks occur during sleep.

When the whole process of sleep NON-REM (Phases One to Four) plus REM sleep is complete, the whole cycle starts again and you experience about four to five of these cycles progressively during the night. As the night progresses, the REM phases become longer and deep-sleep phases gradually become shorter. When morning arrives, the chances of deep sleep are highly unlikely and you spend more time in REM sleep.

Human Growth Hormone Floods the Body During NON-REM

You must remember that during NON-REM (Phase Three to Four: Deep Sleep) is when the anti-ageing Growth Hormone is unleashed into the body. This is a great time as you do not have to do anything because your body is switching on its own natural anti-ageing mechanism. Now, imagine if you never, ever missed your phase of Growth Hormone release – you would have a body that is in the habit of healing itself to look younger. This will explain why sometimes you feel stunningly refreshed after a good night's sleep and have the urge to dress up and make yourself look sexy. You can bet your bottom dollar that that's the night when your body has been able to flood you with Growth Hormone.

I Regularly Miss my Growth Hormone

There is the downside to all this in that many people miss their natural Growth Hormone injection every night. This is because Growth Hormone secretion decreases with age in both sexes. Even though the amount of sleep may not change, the quality does. The problem occurs when you are a habitual sleep offender who sleeps at unpredictable times or, even worse, has very little sleep at all. This is not permitted on the Dr Nirdosh Plan as it is seriously prematurely ageing and also exposes you to medical complications such as high blood pressure, stroke, depression and memory loss. Miss this, and you miss the body's natural recovery phase so it remains full of stress hormones, leaving it in a tired, ageing state. If you continue in this way, I promise you that you will look decades older than you should. Your body will not release melatonin or Growth Hormone optimally, but instead will be encouraged to release bad stress hormones such as insulin and cortisol.

Sleep is vital if you want to anti-age your body and face and discover a sexier new you with a stronger libido. This is only possible if you never miss the deep-sleep phase that gives you vital Growth Hormone: the body still secretes low levels of Growth Hormone through the day and night, but you want the huge Growth Hormone peaks that occur in deep sleep. Let's reintroduce Human Growth Hormone back into your body through sleep. Here are the correct sleep guidelines:

- Avoid alcohol late in the evening as this may initially send you to sleep, but there's a high probability that it will also cause you to wake during the night, so disturbing your sleep cycle.
- Caffeine and stimulants late in the evening will also keep you up late, so avoid them at all costs. These include fizzy drinks, coffee, tea and even hot chocolate – they all contain caffeine.
- Don't take sleeping pills without medical supervision as the consequence of coming off them could lead to full-blown insomnia and other sleep problems.
- Do not go without sleep for long periods as this will cause sleep deprivation and issues such as anxiety, depression or insomnia. When you do feel tired, go to sleep. Try to create some form of routine so your body understands when sleep time has arrived.
- Late meals should be avoided – not only will they make you put on weight, but they'll also give you a burst of energy that you may have to expend, which could keep you up a lot of the night.

For a good night's sleep, make sure that you…

- Always relax one hour before bedtime and do something simple such as reading a book or watching your favourite TV programme.
- Exercise during the day as this helps tire the body, which means you sleep better. Don't exercise too late in the evening

as your body will be racing – working out can be a powerful stimulant.

- Try to address issues that concern you during the day and come to a realistic solution that will not cause you to be thinking late at night. That way, you will not dwell on things and will sleep more peacefully.

- Make sure your room is prepared for sleep and sleep alone. Do not use it as an office, restaurant or cinema-in-one – you get my point. It is for sleep only and your body should know that being in the bedroom means it's time to rest.

- Make love to your partner: being on the plan will refuel your sex drive. Good sex also triggers endorphins so you feel a 'high' and it's also an excellent relaxant.

- Tire your brain – many people engage in physical work, but the brain is not tired. But it needs to be as this is how it enters the deep-sleep phase. If you have not worked your brain during the day, then engage in some intelligent stimulation such as reading, crossword puzzles or even a night class that involves some brain power and coordination – even a sexy salsa dance or Egyptian history lesson! Expanding your mind makes you mentally tired and ready for bed.

- Ensure good sleep hygiene – clean bed covers and fresh nightwear. Consider having a hot relaxing bath before bedtime.

- Eye masks are a good way to help block out any light while sleeping. They are really useful if you are away from home or travelling.

- Ear-plugs are a good way of shutting yourself off from outside noise.
- Playing soothing music can distance you from stressful thoughts and help you to nod off.
- Keep paper and a pen next to your bed. If you wake up in the night and remember a task you have to do the next day, you can scribble it down and then drift off back to sleep without having to worry about how to remember it.

By now you will have realised that sleep is a powerful anti-ageing treatment and, through implementing the rules above, you can regain deep sleep that gives you a massive Human Growth Hormone boost to make your face and body younger.

Chapter 10

Endorphins – The Anti-Ageing High

ENDORPHINS, COMMONLY KNOWN as the feel-good hormones, provide us with a natural high and euphoria. This is the hormone which people in a low state of mind are required to reinstate through natural sources such as exercise, food, laughter and even sexual activities. But for me endorphins are particularly wonderful because they serve a dual purpose – they give us joy and are also a powerful anti-ageing hormone.

WHY WE NEED ENDORPHINS

A rush of endorphins blocks pain and give us an intense, euphoric feeling. Endorphins mimic the actions of the painkillers morphine and cocaine, but are even better as they are naturally present in the human body and are non-addictive analgesics. At some point in our lives, we all suffer pain and Nature's given hormone gift works to block it by providing us with a natural high instead.

When released, endorphins are transported via two channels in the body. Those released by the pituitary gland enter the bloodstream, while those released by nerves in the hypothalamus are transported into the brain and spinal cord. The purpose is to get to the pain receptors fast and obstruct the ache, while producing a feeling of wellbeing in both brain and body. Put simply, the body relies on and needs endorphins to achieve a state of elation to combat physical, mental or emotional pain. Endorphins also help us to defy the ageing process in three important ways, which I will now describe.

Block Cortisol: The Hormone That Causes Stress and Ageing

It has long been documented by medical research that people who are regularly happy not only look younger, but tend to live longer too. A lot of this happiness is down to a healthy flow of natural endorphins. Not only do they block pain but they also block one of the most dangerous hormones in the body that causes ageing: the stress hormone cortisol. In defeating cortisol, the damage that normally ages the body is taken over by endorphins and they work hard to help your body remain young by overriding ageing and stress. This has a major effect on the state of your brain and keeps you mentally content, with your stress under control.

The Cocktail

The Dr Nirdosh Anti-Ageing Body Plan workouts have been developed to provide you with a cocktail of mood enhancers. These are: serotonin, dopamine and adrenaline. Combined with endorphins, they give you a powerful cocktail of feel-good hormones that counteracts any negative feelings and puts the brakes on the ageing system because you will block the hormones that instigate the ageing processes through this unique anti-ageing system.

Superoxide Dismutase (SOD)

This is the most important of the three ways because endorphins have a special capability that helps the human body live longer through the power of antioxidants. Oxygen provides us with life and we need it to live, but a lack of it causes our eventual death. When we breathe in oxygen, it can turn into Superoxide. This is harmful and causes ageing as it damages our inner organs, leading to illness, diseases and death. Endorphins can actually remove Superoxide and neutralise its actions so that the oxygen you breathe no longer causes premature ageing. Endorphins are amazing as they hold the antidote for this process.

HOW THEY WORK

Endorphins facilitate the production of SOD, a special enzyme that the body needs to neutralise the harmful toxicity effects of Superoxide. They keep both body and brain cells healthy through the enhanced action of SOD. This is extremely anti-ageing and gives you the possibility of a younger body and longer life.

HOW TO GET ENDORPHINS BACK INTO YOUR BODY

These are the ways to get endorphins naturally back in your body:

The Dr Nirdosh Anti-Ageing Plan: When you engage in the right kind of physical exercise, the body automatically releases endorphins. The Dr Nirdosh Anti-Ageing exercises help secrete anti-ageing hormones in the body to fend off ageing. My special workouts also activate the brain to unleash a range of feel-good anti-ageing hormones, including serotonin, dopamine, adrenaline and endorphins. Once you start to experience such a high of hormones after a workout, you will never want to stop. The feeling of confidence and sexual attraction as you start to de-age your body will take over your mind. You'll feel such a strong desire for this that it will make you want to step right back into the exercise arena and get those feel-good, anti-ageing hormones going again.

Sex: The hormone that floods the body during sex is endorphin – when you orgasm, your body is flooded with it. This is one of the reasons why the medical profession advises couples to have a healthy sexual relationship: not only does it give you a great feeling when you both orgasm but it also banishes stress and makes demanding situations seem trivial and more manageable. Columbia University did some research and found that having more than 200 orgasms a year can reduce your physiological age by six years – now that's anti-ageing reason enough for some extra laps in the sack!

Chocolate: Yes! It's that good old-fashioned aphrodisiac that we can't wait to get our teeth into and it releases feel-good hormones into the body. Now you must be careful as this is not a passport to stuff yourself, as it will only lead to weight gain, sugar surges and risk of diabetes. Instead, I'm talking about small amounts that give the brain and body a good feeling and help unleash endorphins. The highest value of chocolate is best: at least 80 per cent cocoa solids.

Food: Certain foods can release endorphins; however, please note that these are normally stimulating foods such as wasabi sauce, peppers, chillies and horseradish.

Thrill-givers: I know you'll think I've gone crazy, but what I mean is the kind of thrill that gives sheer excitement. When in thrill-seeking situations, the body normally experiences the 'fight or flight reaction' and this places it in a state of high alert. This is only good in controlled instances as it leads to the secretion of adrenaline (which we don't want all the time because its effect of raising blood pressure, heart rate and stimulating the nervous system puts the body under stress and accelerates ageing if prolonged), as well as masses of endorphins. Such instances include orgasms, rollercoasters at theme parks or watching a scary movie. The immensely exciting feeling that you have while doing these things produces a feeling of ecstasy.

Increase Serotonin Levels: This is not a hormone but a chemical in the brain that is highly documented as a partner of endorphins. It is a neurotransmitter that plays a number of vital roles in the body, including the regulation of sleep habits, body temperature, cardiovascular functionality, mood elevation and appetite control. All these benefits alone could settle the argument that endorphins are important as they aid the body to manufacture serotonin and keep levels healthy, but this is not the reason why we have to address serotonin on the Dr Nirdosh Plan. The sole reason why serotonin is a key player in the body is that it is widely known as the 'happiness chemical', which can help fight depression. Other hormones such as endorphins do a great job in tackling depression and creating the feel-good factor that the body needs, but serotonin flows through the central nervous system and affects nerve impulses in the brain. This makes it a really diverse and responsible transmitter capable of controlling all types of behaviour and traits.

Once you start the Dr Nirdosh Anti-Ageing exercises, the routine will assist your brain to naturally and organically manufacture serotonin so you can have a constant flow of age-reversing hormones, as well as feel-good ones that will quash any low feelings. The amazing thing with serotonin is that, even after you have completed your special anti-ageing exercises, your body continues to release serotonin for up to two days. This is very important as this will programme your body to banish negativity and replace it with positive messages.

Meditation: This increases serotonin levels in the brain even if you only meditate for small amounts of time. The positive thoughts and relaxation effect help increase serotonin levels in the brain and may even enhance Growth Hormone release.

Finally, **smiling and laughter** instantly increase your endorphins levels. Even if you force a smile, it works – so keep smiling! Better still, you may notice the 'high' after an episode of laughter, so engage in fits of laughter at any opportunity you can.

Chapter 11

A Provocative Plan for a Provocative Woman

THE POWER OF sex is highly under-rated. It's a potent anti-ageing remedy and one that the Dr Nirdosh Plan will unleash. Unfortunately, the benefits of a high libido haven't been widely publicised because sex remains a taboo subject, especially where women are concerned, and it has been this way for generations.

Years ago, the orgasmic euphoria of sex was eminent and exploited through undercover images such as the statue of Venus and the Kama Sutra, a guide to nearly every sexual position, including the impossible. Today, we are less inclined to shy away from sex and mainstream celebrities such as Sharon Stone and Demi Moore prove that women can be risqué and still be admired. Contrary to belief, the sexy image that they have is by no means a matter of chance, but comes with a very tactile approach. For years, A-list celebrities have been secretly following the Dr Nirdosh Plan because they know that, to look so steamy, you must have a proven method to ignite sexual fuel within the body. With age, most people suffer a huge loss of sexual hormones and with this the demise of libido and sex appeal. On the plan, however, you will be thrashing this ageism as you follow the A-list way to utter sexiness!

It's great news that old-fashioned stereotypes are fading and at last we are free to talk about sex. Before, it was only men who were allowed to fulfil their sexual desires and the excuse was male testosterone causing men to be on heat. As if women didn't have sexual hormones or tendencies and didn't feel the same arousal! How wrong could they be? Week by week, as we turn back the clock on ageing and restore your body to youth, it will become so engorged with sex hormones that you'll find it impossible to disguise your revitalised desire and sexy new body!

These days, women don't have to prove themselves a virgin on marriage and instead many opt for sexual exploration with a number of partners before they decide to settle down. There's nothing wrong with this and men don't look down at it any more, but actually respect an experienced, independent woman in the same way as women do men. In fact, we will be revelling in this development because the plan has been designed to make you a sexual creature. From the way you dress to how adventurous you are in the bedroom, the 'Dr Nirdosh Way' will make you feel sexually liberated.

A feisty new sexy and flirtatious woman has emerged and what's really important in the 21st century is that females are no longer having sex simply to reproduce, but because they actually enjoy it. As you become sexier on this plan, it will not just be about straightforward intercourse either – the pleasures of foreplay, masturbation and sexual discovery will become super-primed. If you can't recall the sensation and meaning of orgasms, believe me, you will be reminded in an unforgettable way! Get ready to discover your G-spot and prove wrong the sceptics who think women don't get turned on, except the textbook way! Women don't want to always be guided by men – they want to take the plunge, be the leader and indulge in their own wild and wicked sexual fantasies.

Sex is a natural activity for humans, but like ageing it has a certain stigma attached to it and is seen as a no-go area after you reach a certain age. The great thing for women is that age has no relevance now and, far from sex becoming suppressed, the opposite is true. Historically, men were seen as the lucky ones, who can have sex until the day they die, but now so too can women. Our fertility status has also vastly changed opinions as glamorous older celebrity mums such as Madonna confirm that many of us can still successfully reproduce when we're way past 40 and still look hot.

Indeed, the rush to have children before 30 is fast becoming an old-fashioned image. Scientific advances, plus following a healthy lifestyle and advanced medical care, have allowed this to happen and no one is more aware of it than celebrities. And now you have in your hands their secrets to remaining young, sexy and active. On the plan, your fertility system will also see an improvement as you become regenerated, youthful and healthier inside. As many of today's women have decided to give birth a decade or two later than their mothers did, maintaining this fertile quality is vital.

As your confidence increases on the plan, the realisation of what you desire will become clearer so you won't feel so afraid of sexual experimentation or your advancing years. Your bedroom age and body will radiate youth, as you learn to ignore your paper age and accept the new, younger you. This is just the pick-me-up that you'll need in this era of role reversal, whereby older woman are captivating younger men. Once it was older men who would flaunt their youthful beauties, but now 50-plus women can be as attractive as their younger counterparts and have caught the eye of handsome young male prey!

On the plan, we will ensure 20-something girls have some competition on their hands from sexy, alluring experienced women! We are successful in our careers, as well as independent, and with the great sex appeal that the Dr Nirdosh Plan provides, we don't need to be the quiet, controlled secondary partners any more. Throw those thoughts away and welcome a sexually transformed, provocative new you. Move over male supremacy, on the Dr Nirdosh Plan, female domination will triumph! Sexual rebels are arriving, and we're loving it!

SEX IS THE POWER OF YOUTH

All this sexual confidence is not just about freeing women and feeling electric in the bedroom – there's real science to getting high on orgasms. I'm a strong believer in sexually empowering women because there are immense anti-ageing benefits to be drawn from having a healthy and active sexual libido, which are not to be missed. Medically, it is one of the fountains of youth as the chemicals that are released during and after intercourse not only de-age your whole body, but also provide you with an unparalleled level of confidence and youthful essence. This helps improve overall life expectancy, allowing you to live longer.

A Provocative Plan for a Provocative Woman

People often take sex for granted until they hit their early forties because they believe that desire will always be there. It's all well and good, allowing the freedom to be sexy at any age, but, unfortunately, if you do nothing about it, sexual urges can fade with increasing age. This is not just due to boredom or routine, as some sex therapists would have you think, but it's mainly down to chemical changes the body undergoes as a result of sexual-hormone depletion. If we are to keep the ignition going, then we cannot allow sex hormones to dwindle.

When we are younger, we have no such problem. We're fuelled with high levels of testosterone and oestrogen and that's what makes us attractive to others. This high-powered sexual libido, with uncontrollable hormones, is not just part of a natural process to find a suitable partner, it's also a way that the body tells you that it's still virile and agile – and most importantly, young! The hormones manufactured and secreted within the body during the mid-teens right up to the thirties are immensely beneficial as the body releases masses of DHEA (Dehydroepiandrosterone, a vital anti-ageing hormone that works both as a complete entity and when it is broken down into smaller parts – the smaller fragments are then used to make other vital hormones including testosterone and oestrogen), Growth Hormone, testosterone and oestrogen – all powerful anti-ageing hormones that instantly fight off stress and age factors. These power hormones release a sexual surge and large amounts of endorphins to flood the brain with feel-good factors and make our minds and moods dynamic.

The bad news is that, as we age, levels of testosterone and oestrogen rapidly decline because the manufacturing and receptive process of these super sex hormones becomes inefficient. At this point, sexual desire goes haywire and it's not as strong as it was in your teens. This change affects many people mentally. Losing their sexuality makes them feel inadequate. It is not uncommon for people to seek medical help. If you are in a relationship, loss of sexual activity can cause real conflict, especially if one partner's desire has not diminished, but the other's has. This is why medications such as Viagra are now more common, especially for males who see their sex lives shortening with age and HRT common for many menopausal women. This may seem like the only solution but the problem is that you're popping pills to address one issue, while not actually making the body any younger naturally, so it continues to decay and age. So, can it be treated in another way?

Wouldn't you love to defy the natural process of ageing and even regain your sexual drive so you feel sexy again? That's why this six-week programme is a miracle life plan: not only does it make you look younger and teach you how to regain youth through changing your lifestyle, but it also gives you back your sex drive. The Dr Nirdosh Anti-Ageing Plan is the solution that restores your sexuality so you feel like you're back in your teens. But this plan should come with a warning: you will feel so orgasmic that you'll be like a woman let loose or a man re-entering his sexual prime! One of the main reasons why my celebrity clients love this revolutionary plan is that it's more than just anti-ageing for the face and body, but also works to reignite the sex hormones within the body and gives you bucket-loads of sex appeal and youth without the need for pills.

YOUNGER BODY, YOUNGER SEX DRIVE!

Over the next six weeks, you will use this special plan to completely transform your state so that your face, body and sex life radiate youth. This will be achieved by following the four disciplines. As the transition takes place and your body starts to undo ageing right in front of your eyes, you will experience a real change and part of this change is the sexual chemicals in your body. This is one of the true powers of the plan: I call it The Body & Sex Connection.

On the plan, your sex drive will strengthen and you'll feel so sexy and alluring. The point to remember is that this is a special life and body plan that will transform your whole body to become young again by reintroducing anti-ageing hormones. Sex hormones come alive as they are forced to redevelop. Women will learn to fight the menopause and, even after it, recapture their waning sexuality, while men will learn to combat their mid-life-crisis-causing 'Andropause' (the male equivalent of the female menopause). The result is that your libido levels will go through the roof as you rediscover the sex hormones that have a tendency to fade with age, including testosterone, oestrogen and progesterone.

So, let's look at the sex hormones that the plan helps to reintroduce into your body and how we will increase them. These are special hormones that will give you the passport to nights of pleasure, so pay attention!

Testosterone

Throughout your whole life, testosterone plays a key role in aiding your body's youth development and healthy sexuality. The needs and purpose of testosterone change as your body ages and maintaining levels is key. Loss equals ageing and sexual inadequacy.

Testosterone in Males

The male body is composed of androgens, sexual steroids considered to be the male sex hormones, and the most predominant of all is testosterone. This is widely known as the male hormone responsible for male sexual virility. Female bodies do produce testosterone, but nowhere near as much as males. A male body can contain 20 times more testosterone than a female's, which is the reason why it's been publicised that men have more aggression and greater sexual urges than women.

The Teen Years

Throughout your whole life, your body is serviced with testosterone. It is initially responsible for the development of the male sexual organs, including the testes, and provides the body with progressive growth maturation of sexual organs. The actual growth of the penis and scrotum is affected by testosterone during pre-teen years and a deficiency here could mean underdeveloped sexual organs that may not function correctly in further life. Testosterone then goes even further and helps the formation of sperm. With cases of infertility in men on the increase, research has been conducted into whether lower levels of testosterone are responsible, so again this is vital to the development of the male form.

As males enter their teens, testosterone is the hormone that gives the male form its sexual oomph. Sex drive is a major factor and some bodies produce excess testosterone at this time, which can contribute to adverse effects such as acne breakouts and even hair loss. However, normally, the body maintains the required levels.

As males become sexually active in their teens, testosterone levels are at their highest, ensuring they have a healthy and active sex life, with no real medical complications or errors. So in effect, testosterone not only makes the male feel sexy but also allows the correct development of the sex organs in the body. Males who are looking to mate with a female suitor are an indication that sexual function is at its optimum level of functionality. This process enhances male fertility. Libido is just as nature intended, in its true element as testosterone flows round the body in full force. This also means the male body is well equipped to engage in dangerous situations and will withstand traumas, if they should arise.

Testosterone also aids the development of facial hair, deepening the post-pubescent voice, and creates a more muscular body mass frame. It is essential to maintain good levels of testosterone during the teen years to ensure that these natural steroid hormones remain in flourishing quantities within the body. Deficiency can lead to all kinds of serious medical complications, not just loss of desire.

Testosterone in Adulthood

As you grow and enter adulthood, testosterone serves a secondary purpose as it helps further development of the whole body, not just the sex organs. Indeed, testosterone takes a major role and fights hard to defend the body from ageing. It is created in the testes, although a small amount is also produced by the tiny adrenal glands that lie on the kidneys. Testosterone improves overall energy levels, enhances cardiovascular activity and helps the body maintain its vital muscular tissue. This fights off major ageing complications, such as muscular deterioration, to ensure you don't lose your lean body mass. If you do so as a result of declining testosterone levels, your body will start to age rapidly. The loss of muscular fibres sets off a series of activities that change your body composition to have a higher fat ratio. Loss of lean mass and muscle degeneration mean that your body has become seriously weak and under the skin the lost muscle causes sagging and jowls – quite common in inactive middle-aged men. Testosterone loss also leaves the bones vulnerable to breaks and causes moodiness, the mind is less sharp, stamina and strength reduces and ageing is accelerated throughout the whole body. This snowball effect will carry on unless it is interrupted and halted. As you can tell, it is essential to conserve testosterone in the body if you want to remain young and active.

The problem of testosterone degradation starts as early as the late twenties, so, even when you think you are at your optimum level at the age of 30, internally you have already begun to lose this mighty anti-ageing hormone. It shows no signs of letting up, with levels of loss year on year increasing as you go through decade after decade. This can be attributed to ageing; however, what you must realise is that this is not just a natural progression that you have to abide by because it brings with it serious medical problems.

The brain is directly affected by low levels of testosterone because it no longer receives the free flow it once did and this reduces its capabilities and alertness. Known complications include loss of attention span and ailing memory, so you may suffer bouts of recall loss. If this progresses further, symptoms could result in a diagnosis of Alzheimer's disease. Testosterone is also needed to allow healthy red blood cell production and to preserve bone strength. Another key factor is the loss of sexual functionality in the gonads (sex organs), reduced endurance and no real need to be engaged in sexual activities. This is a major problem for many men and relationships: not only do they feel they are no longer able to sense stimulation, but they also feel that they are letting their partner down. Many males may immediately suffer a real lack of confidence and feel they are inadequate in the eyes of society; also that they are ageing. In effect, the loss of testosterone has placed their body in a degenerative, ageing state.

As the pressure mounts and the loss becomes greater, there is every possibility that the male may suffer erectile dysfunction. This can lead to a myriad of complications within a relationship. Lack of sexuality can make the male fall into deep depression, requiring medical help to treat the condition. The body no longer has a posture composed of a strong and firm stance. Instead, as the body weakens, posture becomes a slouch. At this stage, the body is ageing rapidly and the chances of regaining sexual youth may be a distant memory.

It's Not Just for Men!

While females do not have the same amount of testosterone as men, contrary to belief, they still have this male-named hormone, normally about one-seventh of the amount of a man's. Women too will lose testosterone with age; the collapse works around a similar principle, but is more geared towards the ovaries. Likewise, testosterone in females contributes to sex drive and maintenance of muscle strength. It helps fight muscle degeneration and sexual libido that appears to have gone AWOL.

Female testosterone is produced in the ovaries as well as the adrenal glands. As this hormone loses its prime, it can lead to the same feelings of rejection and lack of sexual desire as males going through the Andropause experience. Another complication that directly affects sex drive in women is the menopause. After the menopause, women's bodies take on a different form – they have a body composition largely made up of fat and very little muscle tissue. Most women relate these changes to loss of the female sex hormones oestrogen and progesterone, while the significance of testosterone affecting sexual status is often totally dismissed. The Dr Nirdosh Plan tackles this huge medical mistake as its natural hormonal replacement therapy effect includes boosting levels of testosterone, too.

The menopause is largely down to lost oestrogen and progesterone, but testosterone is also a vital element of female ageing. During this time, elasticity is hampered and collagen levels fall. Skin becomes lose, limp, dry and creased while the face looks sagged. The body feels soft and lumpy, and weight piles on more easily. Women want to look and feel sexy, but they don't because their levels of testosterone and the other female sex hormones, oestrogen and progesterone, drop. Trying to remain sexy and youthful may seem like a world away, but not on this plan!

Clearly, a drop in testosterone poses a risk of ageing and allows damage to the body. Up until now, you may not have been aware of the importance of this hormone in women, but, if you don't take action, then you will surely say goodbye to looking and feeling sexually primed.

THE ANTI-AGEING BODY PLAN

The Dr Nirdosh Anti-Ageing Plan gives you back your sexuality by helping to increase your levels of testosterone in two ways. It will aid the body to naturally reproduce and increase levels of testosterone. A major driving force of the plan is to elevate anti-ageing hormones and one of the disciplines does this through a new technique of anti-ageing exercises. Not only will the exercises that you embark on over the next six weeks make your body look sexier and younger, but they will also revive the natural anabolic steroid hormone (testosterone) within your body so that you can appear hot and youthful again.

Not only that, but you'll begin to feel yourself aroused and foxy, almost as if you are going back in time! As the testosterone runs through your bloodstream and floods your organs via the special Dr Nirdosh Anti-Ageing exercises, your sexuality will come alive. The highly skilled, specialised movements will encourage a natural secretion of testosterone. This testosterone enhancement also helps to define firmer face and body contours as your lean muscle tissue increases to give a 'nip and tuck' look. Finally, you'll discover how to regain your sex appeal!

YOUTH PILLS

The Dr Nirdosh Anti-Ageing Supplement Plan will aid the body to naturally reproduce and increase levels of testosterone. You will need to implement this as part of your anti-ageing supplement prescription, as described in Chapter 8, and you will be required to take what I call 'youth pills'. Certain groups of these are predominantly composed to provoke the natural manufacture of testosterone.

Once you have implemented both these disciplines into your life, you will start to see the change in your body shape and truly realise what it feels like to have a high libido. The change will take six weeks, but in that time your body will show signs of youth and plentiful testosterone will help awaken your sexual organs. You'll not only look hot and shapely, but also feel damn sexy!

This is a great stride forward as your body is signalling to you that it has become young and healthy again and is back in an anti-ageing youthful mode rather than a downward spiral of serious medical complications.

THE OTHER FEMALE SEX HORMONES
Oestrogen

This is the main female sex hormone that plays an important role in the sexual development of women. It is a complex hormone within the body which differs before and after the female menopause. Made in small amounts by the adrenal glands, most oestrogen is actually produced by the ovaries. It controls the sexual reproductive system within the female body. When a female is in the process of becoming pregnant or trying to have a baby, it is oestrogen that makes this possible. Oestrogen helps protect the female body against endometrial cancer; excess, however, may cause oestrogen-driven tumours of the breast.

The Teen Years

During puberty years, oestrogen assists the development of the female breasts and ovaries. It also allows the body to reproduce and develop periods (menorrhea). You can imagine that, if a female body develops without the correct amounts of oestrogen, then it will never have the ability to fall pregnant. Like most hormones, oestrogen is transported into the bloodstream and then attaches to cell receptors all over, including the nervous system, blood vessels, bones and even the brain.

Oestrogen in Adulthood

The function of oestrogen is not just limited to the sex organs of the female body, although this is one of its main purposes. It has a wide host of other benefits, determining many health outcomes. Oestrogen helps maintain healthy bones, keeping them dense and strong. It also works to elevate HDL (good) cholesterol and reduce levels of LDL (bad) cholesterol. Oestrogen also has a feel-good factor associated to it because its levels impact on the brain to help it remain in a youthful and positive state. It helps banish conditions such as depression, but the reason why it is really special to females is because it is also a powerful anti-ageing hormone as well as a sex hormone.

Oestrogen works to maintain skin collagen and elasticity in the female body. This helps facial skin remain uplifted and sag-free. When levels are abundant, you will have a glowing, dewy and plumped complexion. Skin elasticity remains fruitful, thus preventing skin ageing, collagen is buoyant and the accumulative anti-ageing effect of oestrogen results in thicker facial skin. It also helps keep skin moist and lubricated, and prevents the 'droop', helping the frame of skin to stay uplifted. If you want your face to fight the ageing process, maintaining healthy levels of oestrogen is paramount. It allows a woman to feel sexy and provides a face and body that resists age-related decay.

The problem is that, as we age, oestrogen levels decline: for women the changes experienced by the body are truly life changing, mentally as well as physically. One of the biggest causes of this change is the menopause, a phase that causes the female body to rapidly lose the supply of sex hormones, including oestrogen, progesterone and testosterone. The biggest medical change to occur is the type of oestrogen that your body produces before and after the menopause. Pre-menopause oestrogen is a combination of three small hormones: oestradiol, oestrone and oestriol. Oestradiol is the driving force in pre-menopausal oestrogen hormones but, when the female body experiences the menopause, oestrone becomes the main part. When this chemical imbalance happens, a decline in oestrogen levels occurs and dramatically alters the body. Symptoms include the following:

- Skin becomes drier and/or thinner
- Hair starts to thin
- Skin sags and wrinkles
- The body becomes prone to brittle bones and heart attacks

- Weight is more readily gained
- Abdominal, hip and thigh region fat accumulation dominates
- Sex drive vanishes
- Vaginal dryness occurs
- Memory and mood problems surface
- Hot flushes and sleep problems occur
- Enhanced risk of stroke.

These are all indicators that the body is ageing and this is why some women opt for HRT to try to beat the menopause. The physical changes are dramatic and cause a sudden difference from a youthful state to a mature one. The Dr Nirdosh Anti-Ageing Plan gives you back your sexuality by increasing your levels of oestrogen in three ways, as follows.

The Anti-Ageing Body Plan

The Dr Nirdosh Anti-Ageing Body Plan will aid the body to naturally reproduce and increase levels of oestrogen. Over the next six weeks, specialist movements will be incorporated into your routine to help elevate sex hormones, including oestrogen. As your levels of oestrogen increase on this plan, your body will become younger and sexier. Libido levels will soar and you'll experience your sexuality being set on fire again. The term 'feeling orgasmic' could be classed as an understatement! This younger body will become competent again and equipped to block ageing. As this injection of youth occurs, the body does a U-turn and lets the sex hormones run riot as it assumes that it's back in its teens again. Get ready to rediscover a younger, sexier you!

The Anti-Ageing Nutrition Plan

The Dr Nirdosh Anti-Ageing Nutrition Plan will aid the body to naturally reproduce and increase levels of oestrogen. Special foods, including soya and yam, help elevate oestrogen. The plan encourages the consumption of phytoestrogen-rich foods, such as soya and yam, as they have properties known to mimic the action of oestrogen. For women, incorporating this into the food plan during and after the menopause is essential.

The Anti-Ageing Supplement Plan

The Dr Nirdosh Anti-Ageing Supplement Plan aids the body to naturally reproduce and increase levels of oestrogen. Specific supplements will be used to enhance oestrogen sources for women experiencing the menopause or having passed this mid-life condition. The body will be fed dedicated supplements as a natural form of HRT drawn from soya, yam and other oestrogen-mimicking or provoking ingredients. In this way, you can avoid the dangerous side effects that may occur with regular HRT and still benefit from the oestrogen-enhancing effect of natural hormonal boosters.

Progesterone

As well as oestrogen, the female body has another special sex hormone linked directly to the female reproductive system and, if this hormone flows with abundance, you can really experience the joys of greater sexual stimulation and pleasure. Progesterone is the secretive sex hormone. This hormone makes the female body fertile and is responsible for preparing the uterus to have babies. It also helps female breasts take on their soft, rounded shape as oestrogen dominance can makes them fibrous.

Progesterone can also help evade oestrogen-driven cell division seen in certain cancers, such as breast cancer. In the brain and nervous system it has neuro-protective effects, while in the body it induces anti-inflammatory action throughout, so it's a vital function to protect against ageing. The problem is that most women do not know enough about this hormone and the powers it holds to unleash sexual juices. So how does it work?

After childbirth or the menopause, most women lose their sexual desire or sex appeal and again deem this as a consequence of ageing. They think that they have to accept that a sexual low is something all women of a certain age will experience. But this myth is so untrue and, if the progesterone levels are corrected, then you have every possibility of unlocking the key to that hidden G-spot and saying hello to more years of happy, orgasmic sex!

The Teen Years

As the female body develops in its teens, it goes through natural changes and developments that prepare it for womanhood. The two main hormones that help this evolution process to take place are oestrogen and progesterone. At this stage, the female form takes on everlasting changes that will determine its womanly shape.

Although women don't realise it, not only are these hormones shaping the way their body looks and performs, but they are also doing something far more clever and essential to the future of the human race. Once they have completed their task of successful puberty transition, they move on to phase two and become the hormones associated with the female reproductive system. As well as oestrogen, the ovaries produce the sex hormone progesterone. This control is regulated by the brain hypothalamic-pituitary system, which monitors hormone levels by a negative feedback loop. The clever signalling tells the body when and which hormones need to be released, which assists healthy ovaries to regulate a woman's reproductive and menstrual cycle.

This is a unique change as the female sex hormones now work to prepare for ovulation and to reproduce on a fairly monthly cycle. Just before and right after ovulation, progesterone and oestrogen levels rise massively to prepare the female vagina and uterus for conception and a high sexual desire is experienced at this time. If fertilisation does not take place, then levels decline and menstruation occurs. Imbalances of these hormones just before a period are thought to be behind PMS (Pre-menstrual Syndrome): moodiness, bloated stomach, skin breakouts, tiredness, irritability, impaired thinking, breast tenderness/swelling and food cravings.

Progesterone in Adulthood

This sexual time in a woman's life is an amazing feat as little effort is required from the female due to all the sexual juices that naturally flow through her body. Progesterone levels are good and the female is ready to mate with a suitor. This makes a woman feel sexy and ready to take action! The feeling that you experience during these years can be satisfaction at its heightened state and emulating this sexual high can only take effect in later years if you take measures to sustain your sexuality.

At these high moments, the vaginal wall is lubricated and ready to orgasm during sex. It will provide feelings of satisfaction and give you confidence about your body. The breasts become more sensitive to touch sensations, libido levels go through the roof and sexual juices flow direct to the pelvic section, allowing your sex life to be at its best ever.

Remember, the purpose is to give you the sexual tools required for successful pregnancy so the hormones make your body look forward to sex. At this point, progesterone does another amazing thing. A well-fertilised egg allows pregnancy to proceed and the hormones to take on a new role. Now the female hormones are all directed towards achieving a successful pregnancy and flow at even higher rates. Furthermore, a new hormone – Human Chorionic Gonadotrophin (HCG) – comes into the equation to make pregnancy possible. This hormone is crucial as it stimulates the ovaries to maintain the corpus luteum and continue producing exceptionally high levels of progesterone, so the uterus remains in a condition to allow foetal growth. Oestrogen production also carries on throughout to sustain pregnancy, so both these sex hormones remain at a high level. That's why some women feel so energetic and sexy during their pregnancy and have a strong desire to continue having sex while carrying, as their body just bursts at the seams with sexual stamina! And the benefits don't stop there: pregnancy alone can give women stunning anti-ageing benefits because the increased levels help skin to look glowing, fuller and more beautiful than ever. Also, increased levels of progesterone can make your hair noticeably stronger and thicker.

Fight the Decline

After pregnancy the body takes an almost automatic U-turn, which is when losses start to become apparent. Decline in the sex hormones creates a loss of sexual libido. It is needed, however, as the quick fall in progesterone allows the body to produce milk (lactation) so the mum can breastfeed her newborn.

The problem is that progesterone is also associated with mood and, as this drops, the mood of the female changes drastically. It has been known to be a root cause of the symptoms of postnatal depression. In fact, the whole change that the body goes through at this stage is quite dramatic: the womb goes back to its original size, blood flow minimises and the pelvic muscles relax. It happens almost instantly and contributes to the loss of sexual desire as well as other medical conditions.

There is another time when the female body goes through a sudden loss of sex hormones and that is during the menopause. The ovaries slowly start to produce hormones less effectively, so levels of oestrogen and progesterone diminish. This brings the onset of symptoms of the menopause such as hot flushes, night sweats and also enhanced risk of heart disease and osteoporosis. As progesterone and oestrogen develop mainly in the ovaries, once these sex organs don't function properly any more, then the hormonal synthesis sharply falls. At this stage, it is common for the sexual juices to completely dry out, leaving women feeling totally sexless. The desire to have sex will vanish and, even if you have sex, it can be quite painful because of the vaginal dryness. You might describe this as being well and truly the beginning of the demise of female sexiness.

The reality is that most people do not know about sex hormones and the possibility of regeneration, so they accept the symptoms and sufferings. They do not realise that you can bring them back and regain your sex drive to enjoy a fruitful love life again that is just as good as it was in your teens. The amazing thing is that with this anti-ageing plan you will not only learn how to regain your sexiness, but also how to make it more electric than in your teens! The Dr Nirdosh Anti-Ageing Plan gives you back your sexuality by increasing your levels of progesterone in two ways, as follows.

The Anti-Ageing Body Plan

The Dr Nirdosh Anti-Ageing Body Plan aids the body to naturally reproduce and increase levels of progesterone. The way this will happen is like oestrogen. As your body changes shape and you work hard using the special hormone-boosting Anti-Ageing Body Plan, your hormones start to elevate internally and this includes increased levels of progesterone. The special discipline of the plan makes this possible as you engage in unique movements developed to flood the body with anti-ageing chemicals, including the two female sex hormones: oestrogen and progesterone.

As you transform your body to become younger, the hormones will reappear internally. This will not only enable you to look decades younger, but you'll also feel decades sexier. Your sexual juices will become free flowing so you feel aroused again.

Your vaginal wall will be lubricated and you'll crave sex. When you do have sex, be warned: you will experience orgasmic sex better than it was in your youth years. The heightened sex hormones will make you feel sexy and allow your body to behave as if it is young again. Your body shape will become sexier and you'll feel engorged with sexual desire!

The Anti-Ageing Nutrition Plan

The Dr Nirdosh Anti-Ageing Nutrition Plan consists of foods that will aid the body to naturally boost levels of anti-ageing hormones. Foods on the plan trigger youth and beauty by helping the body to enhance production of the necessary hormones. This nutritional food plan will help to elevate your levels of progesterone. So super boost your sex drive and elevate the hormones inside your body to transform yourself into a born-again sex machine. The following tips will help you achieve mind-blowing orgasms.

Elevate progesterone with these foods:

- Nuts and seeds
- Avocados
- Olive oil
- Lean dairy produce (usually taken from pregnant cows), such as low-fat cheese, low-fat yoghurt and skimmed milk.

Pelvic-Floor Exercise

To strengthen and tighten your vaginal wall so that you can feel penetration and increase sexual pleasure, incorporate this special sex exercise developed to tighten pelvic muscles. When you have sex, you will experience unbelievable orgasms. The Pelvic-Floor Exercise tones the region that becomes loose over the years after having babies or as the menopause approaches. It will also encourage bladder control to return, stopping leaking urine issues, and give you sexy, hot orgasms.

Let's start by locating the pelvic muscles. Imagine you are peeing and have to stop halfway. The muscles that halt the urine flowing out are the pelvic-floor muscles, which stretch from the front of your genitals all the way back to the anal triangle.

Now sit in a chair and separate your legs so there's a gap between your knees. Clench your pelvic muscles. Hold for 10 seconds and then release. Repeat and do 10 more reps this time. When you have finished your first set, do two more sets. In total you will do three sets with 10 repetitions per set, as below:

- One set = 10 reps (hold each rep for 10 seconds and then release)
- Do three sets altogether.

As you become more experienced, you can do more and more sets throughout the day and learn how to give yourself an out-of-this-world orgasm!

The Pelvic-Floor Exercise works to:

- Tighten your vaginal wall
- Restore vaginal tissue

- Increase sensation of sexual pleasure
- Aid in the discovery of orgasmic female ejaculation
- Strengthen muscles
- Halt accidental peeing
- Train your body for longer sex sessions
- Make you feel sexy, confident and much more sensitive to sexual penetration.

The Squat Pelvic Exercise

The next exercise to help you experience mind-blowing orgasms is the squat thrust. Stand in a squat position and clench your pelvic-floor muscles. From an upright position, squat all the way down until your legs are parallel to the floor (if you can go that far, otherwise only go as low as possible to avoid injury). Do the same amount of reps as for the first pelvic-floor exercise. This is the second stage and an advanced movement that helps restore sexiness and orgasmic status in women.

REDISCOVER THE WONDERS OF SEX

Lack of sleep causes the libido to go down so you must ensure that you do not deprive yourself of it. The fatigue makes the body unable to lift itself and feel sexy – it just won't have the energy.

Remember, today's modern women are enjoying sex in later years and it's no longer taboo to do so. The benchmark seems to be set by celebrities and trendsetters such as Raquel Welch and Sophia Loren who boast that they are still basking in a love of good sex, which they attribute to daily exercising and good diets.

They look sexy and are not afraid to voice their joy in having lots of sex.

These women take the necessary steps to ensure they remain sexually virile. Like everything in life, you have to work at things to make the magic happen and, in this case, if you really want to rediscover the wonders of sex in your later years, just add the above tips to your repertoire and relish the thought that, six weeks from now, you will not only look younger, but you'll also have a sex drive to match. You may find yourself so sexually active that younger lovers you encounter may find it hard to keep pace with you! This should make you feel excited and orgasmic even before sex happens. One thing these A-list icons have in common is that they are renowned for their ever-changing looks. They know that, as soon as they stop resembling a sex symbol, their careers will be easily overtaken by younger women waiting in the wings, so they dare not let this happen.

You now have the secret anti-ageing plan with everything you need to experience an orgasmic lifestyle, so use it wisely and love the journey. Your body will release post-orgasmic endorphins so your confidence levels soar and you'll ooze sex! Welcome back your new best friend – your G-spot!

Enjoying a fulfilled sex life is important because it boosts your confidence and you feel young and pleasured. Here are a few final tips:

- Make time for regular sex, even if you have a busy lifestyle, and keep your relationship exciting – don't let it fall into a boring routine. Be spontaneous, flirty and mischievous with your partner. Always take measures to keep your relationship fresh.

- It's important you are both fine-tuned into turning each other on. If you look good, you will feel better, so wear sexy clothes, make innuendos and sexual eye contact when out in public or around the home.

- If you have children or other people living with you, make sure you set a time to go to the bedroom and have a sex-filled night without interference.

- Don't rush into having full-blown sex straight away. Teasing and engaging in foreplay is crucial to enhancing sexual desire and unleashing juices. Spend time enjoying this and you will feel unbelievably excited. Enjoy the build-up as much as the act itself.

- Be erotic and sexually experimental. Enjoy new positions, touch sexually and climax with freedom. Let yourself go and totally trance your mind into a sexy zone. Ooze confidence when naked. After all, you've followed the plans!

- Be confident about your new younger body and exploit what you enjoy sexually. Control and power is extremely alluring, so lead the way forward and don't always wait for him. Be a temptress!

Chapter 12

The New You is Waiting in the Wings!

NOW THERE'S NO excuse whatsoever not to take action. You have the power and knowledge to age-reverse your body to transform yourself into a new, younger and sexier self. So, take action and don't miss this opportunity to acquire your dream body and younger face. Unveiling a new 'to die for' body which look decades younger and a face which is much more youthful will only be the start of your change as these are the drastic results you can achieve in just six small weeks. I am certain that, once you realise that my plan reprogrammes your body to become younger every day, then you will make this a lifestyle and at that stage you will start to really love your life.

You embarked on this journey in the hope of unlocking the secrets that will give you back youth and beauty and now you have that information in the palm of your hands. The human body wasn't made to age rapidly, but, if it is left dormant, it will.

Our current lifestyle is centred round doing all the wrong things and engaging in vices that damage the body's age-defence barrier, which in turn encourages premature ageing. The Dr Nirdosh Plan changes and defeats this. With the plan, you will discover the major anti-ageing defenders and incorporate the secrets into your life. This enables your body to block ageing and reverse the ageing clock so that you can have a body which is healing and fixing itself to correct age-inflicted damage, while flooding you with youth.

The Dr Nirdosh Anti-Ageing Plan was devised in my darkest hours as a junior doctor fighting against the elements of long shifts, poor nutrition, sleep deprivation, depression and premature ageing. This led to the creation of the groundbreaking, age-reversing body plan widely circulating in celebrity circles, as they too wanted an exit strategy from the elements of ageing. Naturally, they did not want to appear aged and haggard in front of their fans and so they requested the Dr Nirdosh Anti-Ageing Plan, so that they had a solution to help them overcome this. Now you too have that solution and can look forward to a younger, more sexier you that defies ageing. The amazing thing is that the Dr Nirdosh Plan promises quick-fix results and in just six short weeks you will experience such wondrous changes and finally gain the younger body and uplifted face of your former youth and beauty.

COUGARS AND SWOFTIES – THEY'RE TALKING ABOUT YOU!

With such media presence daily about the benefits of becoming older and unleashing your sexy alter-ego, as soon as you hit your senior years, it's no wonder that such new terms as female 'cougars' (women with younger toy-boy boyfriends) or SWOfties (single women over 50) have surfaced. We live in a time-savvy generation and the way to keep happy, sane and accepted with social interaction is not to disown these terms as silly fads but rather to embrace and understand them. The Dr Nirdosh Plan helps you reinvent yourself with the confidence to know that you have the single most complete anti-ageing body plan in your hand that allows you to remain always young and sexy, no matter what the latest trend dictates.

ADVANCED SCIENCE = ADVANCED YEARS!

Scientifically, doctors and laboratory technicians are advancing and forever pushing the boundaries to find those ever-elusive medical breakthroughs that help humans counteract the damage that hamper our bodies' immunity and ability to function. The one thing that seems to grab everyone's attention when these findings are published is the ability to live longer by readjusting your lifestyle. The Dr Nirdosh Anti-Ageing Plan complements these new findings and has been specifically created to work on this basis so that you instantly start to internally tune your body to automatically remain in a youthful and ageless state. The plan helps to transform the body not only to look sexier but also to live longer with a more fruitful and happy existence, mentally, physically and sexually.

Key components must be included into our daily lives to ensure that we maximise what the body is given and reap the benefits to remain in a strong, youthful and healthy state. These components include antioxidants, which defend against reactive oxygen species and slow down ageing; vitamins, which deliver essential nutrients that the body can't manufacture itself and allow it to gain stronger immunity; peptides, as they regulate cell growth and control collagen activity in the skin, plus a huge spectrum of vital macro- and micronutrients the body needs, such as protein and EFAs. The plan that you have delivers all these; however, there is a vital missing component in the chain and that is the link that the Dr Nirdosh Plan has created. It's also probably the most important one of all: anti-ageing hormones!

You now have the ultimate anti-ageing plan with the added missing component that the body needs to achieve age-reversing miracles.

IT'S PROBABLY YOUR HORMONES

Hormones, as you now know, are the golden ticket in aiding your body to reinject youth and beauty, as they have the ability to help you readjust from an ageing soft, degenerating, wrinkly state to a strong, upright, muscular, sexy, taut and defined body with a younger face in just six weeks. Left alone, the bad hormones that instigate ageing in adults will flourish and this leads to visual age defects such as deep wrinkles on the face, turkey neck and skin sagging, combined with a body that suffers saggy, bat-winged arms, fat accumulation and premature skin-cell death. Now you can alter the route from the path to destruction. You can defy this preconceived ageing pattern, the pattern so many men and women deem inevitable. Instead, implement the four disciplines of the Dr Nirdosh Plan into your life and in just six weeks watch your body start to transform as the new hormonal flurry forces it to become young again.

SIX WEEKS TO A NATURAL FACE-LIFT

Finally, you will understand what it feels like to look in the mirror and be happy with your reflection because one of the plan's main components is to work directly on the facial skin layers to heal the face so that a younger one can emerge. This is done both externally and internally, and we target the age concerns head-on so that, at the end of the six weeks, you will have noticeable results that boost skin-healing and skin-lifting properties.

Nothing is left to chance: through feeding the skin with vital nutrients, anti-ageing molecules, firming ingredients and hormones over the next six weeks, the face must alter. Welcome to the natural Dr Nirdosh face-lift! The reason why your face is capable of a natural lift is simply because you are no longer starving it of the killer components that it needs to implement change. Your skin famine has ended!

SIX WEEKS TO A NATURAL BODY-LIFT

One of the most obvious and dramatic changes that you will notice over the six-week period is how your body transforms. You will be targeting the whole body in sections and will achieve your goals by following the strict Dr Nirdosh Plan. Age reversal will be substantial, as will weight loss. Not only will you lose weight but also you'll replace the lost weight with new sexier curves and a younger, tauter frame. The amazing thing is that, even though you may be training for only 20 minutes a day, the change is so dramatic.

By following this brand-new doctor-developed special 20-minute exercise programme, you will easily drop more than two dress sizes and essentially tighten all the loose saggy bits, while eliminating fat and reversing the body's ageing mechanism. The initial plan is for just six weeks and, in that short space of time, you will adjust your body to promote youth internally by working on elevating the youth chemicals within.

Followed correctly, the plan will make you look decades younger compared to your real age. You will feel your muscles tone up and your skin tighten to leave a sexy new you with taut and slender curves that you will be dying to show off. After the Dr Nirdosh introductory six-week plan, you'll discover that this is a lifestyle you will not want to give up and you'll feel the urge to carry on. It's easy to do and developed so you can slot it into your daily routine without turning your life upside down. Rather than just incorporating it as a short-term quick fix, I want you to make it a lifestyle so that you can learn to love those killer sexy curves – always!

YOU SEXY THING!

The plan floods sex appeal back into your life in just six weeks. Who wants to become younger but not have youthful, sexy ways? The age-reversing miracle plan makes the body younger all round and your sexual juices will be flowing so your libido levels come alive. After you have completed your transformation, you will notice how you become far more alluring to the opposite sex. Even though you may presently have lost all desire or sexual urges, rest assured the drought is about to break!

The six weeks spent on the plan reintroduce vital sex hormones that decline with age. Having these sex hormones flowing around your body makes you feel like a love-struck teenager again. You'll feel sexy and desire sex as the hormones create this lust. The plan has been known to cause couples to be at it like the proverbial rabbits, so you have been warned!

PROGRESSIVELY YOUTHFUL

If you are to reverse ageing and reinject youth into your body, will the Dr Nirdosh Plan make you live longer? The plan will fix decades of age damage and, if it can do this in just six short weeks, what happens if you follow it for the next six years? The result is that you will have stimulated the body's ability not only to look younger but to live longer, too. As your body slows down its ageing clock, it also slows down the rate at which you age and deteriorate and so increases the ability to live longer. So, yes, this will help you to live longer, too.

But the Dr Nirdosh Plan is much more clever and complex than this and to simply leave it to chance would not be accurate. I want to ensure you live longer, so I've taken it a step further and purposely set in motion the steps to activate a super-special gene that we all have, but is rarely turned on. This gene was highly important to our ancestors as it came into play when they needed to survive on small rations. Since humans have no need to fight for survival as our ancestors did, the gene is normally a dormant one that plays little or no part in our lives, but has amazing powers. SIRT 1 has the ability to help us to live longer.

From day one, the Dr Nirdosh Plan activates the longevity gene. Over the next six weeks, SIRT 1 is the link that allows your body to evolve: as you become younger and look younger, you also help the body to live longer. With all facets of the plan implemented at once, you could help yourself to live up to two decades longer – that's 20 extra years on this planet!

The Dr Nirdosh Plan is the first-ever anti-ageing programme whereby you will notice your body and face become progressively youthful. Yes, you heard me correctly – see yourself becoming younger! You have in your hands the tools to alter your biological age, so you can learn to ignore your real age and live up to your new, younger-than-you image. You'll enjoy seeing yourself look so hot. Anyway, why should you worry about your age if your body is transforming in front of your eyes and you are beginning to feel more youthful and alive as the days pass? This is happening because the plan ensures that your body is equipped to avoid making you older and to fill that void by manufacturing youth – naturally. The overflow of youth will feed your body with youth-induced hormones that will take over the damaging molecules.

Getting used to the plan will soon seem like common practice and you'll love looking at the new and improved you, but let me remind you that being on the six-week plan means that you're a truly unique individual as it is usually only prescribed to celebrities. They know my hormones plan holds the key to unlocking the secrets of de-ageing and, if you gorge the body with the good anti-ageing hormones, you can enhance its ability to become young again. Now you can do this, too.

Undo ageing and enjoy the increased amounts of youth in your body composed of special anti-ageing hormones including: Growth Hormone, testosterone, oestrogen, endorphins and DHEA. This will dampen and override the bad ageing hormones in your body, including the danger hormones that cause premature and accelerated ageing: cortisol, insulin and excess adrenaline.

Using the four Dr Nirdosh disciplines, you have the blueprint of the number-one all-natural face- and body-lift. Simply by following this plan, you will have learned how important each of the four disciplines is and how they work on different parts of the body using the underlying principle of boosting anti-ageing hormones. The four steps have been coordinated to fit into your schedule, whether you are a busy working professional or a home mum racing around kids. Plan in advance as this allows you to stay on the programme and follow it with ease.

The best times for you to tackle each discipline are as follows:

- Dr Nirdosh Anti-Ageing Body Plan: Morning or early evening.
- Dr Nirdosh Anti-Ageing Nutrition Plan: Throughout the day as your daily eating plan.
- Dr Nirdosh Anti-Ageing Skincare Plan: Application twice daily, morning and night.
- Dr Nirdosh Anti-Ageing Supplement Prescription: Regular intervals, around mealtimes throughout the day.

A VISION OF POSITIVITY AND RESULTS

The results will be forthcoming – even after your initial sessions and treatments, you'll see the difference. At this stage envisage the change and do not hold back. Up until now you may not have had the killer plan that you feel would give you the results you expect, but now you do. This is the most complete anti-ageing plan used by celebrities to get their face and body quickly back in shape.

THE ONE-MINUTE VISION

Close your eyes and imagine how you would like to look. Look at your new face and your body. Imagine others looking at you and commenting on how great you look. Visualise how the wrinkles and lines on your face are evaporating. Look at your face and how plump your skin looks as you have worked hard to naturally establish collagen levels. Imagine yourself looking in the mirror and seeing the bags under your eyes become less puffy and crow's feet diminish as your skin heals; they are not as swollen and sore as they looked before. Look at the colour of your complexion – see how vibrant it is, how it glows with youth and radiance. Feel the skin under your neck tighten and your jowls start to uplift again. Love looking at yourself and enjoy experiencing a natural face-lift that you have made possible.

Now think of your body and how much it has transformed in such a short amount of time. Look at how much fat you have lost, how much leaner you look – those sexy curves that you've acquired are so hot that you can't help but show them off! Be impressed with yourself, at how you have lost weight and tightened that saggy loose skin. Commend yourself: you've worked hard for those newly defined, shapely muscles. Finally, think how much younger and sexier you look on the plan. Also, how easy it is. Even when it seems demanding, imagine laughing it off and simply sticking to the plan with ease.